Vocational Training in General Dental Practice

A handbook for trainers

Raj Rattan
BDS MFGDP DipMDE

Forewords by
Penelope Vasey
and
Ian Waite

Radcliffe Medical Press

Radcliffe Medical Press Ltd
18 Marcham Road
Abingdon
Oxon OX14 1AA
United Kingdom

www.radcliffe-oxford.com
The Radcliffe Medical Press electronic catalogue and online ordering facility.
Direct sales to anywhere in the world.

British Library Cataloguing in Publication Data

A catalogue record for this book is available from the British Library.

ISBN 1 85775 232 5

Typeset by Action Publishing Technology Ltd, Gloucester
Printed and bound by TJ International Ltd, Padstow, Cornwall

Contents

Foreword

Since its inception in 1977, vocational training (VT) in dentistry has been constantly evolving. As change in all spheres of life accelerates, and the use of information technology becomes commonplace, the value of a written volume such as this may seem questionable. It is several years since Raj Rattan compiled his first handbook, based on his experiences as a VT Adviser, and this latest offering is in response to countless requests from Trainers for an updated version. The ethos of VT is still the same, with the needs of the Vocational Dental Practitioner (VDP) at its heart. Since the introduction of mandatory VT in 1993, internal structuring, monitoring and guidance have been developed to provide as relevant and high-quality training as possible.

External forces have also produced change, as we have adapted guidance to comply with the law and emulate best practice for adult education.

Every Trainer will recognise the need that occasionally arises rapidly to access information, and this handbook will provide such a resource: either you will find the answer to your query, or it will direct you to an appropriate source of information.

Whilst liaison with the Adviser and Postgraduate Dean will always be crucial in the event of problems arising, to reach for a handbook with so much practical advice will provide instant support. To those Trainers experiencing a smooth ride during the VT year, it is always good to have confirmation that you are 'doing it right'.

Both new and experienced Trainers will find this handbook useful. The sections on Trainer selection, rôle and responsibilities and selection of a VDP bring even the most experienced trainers up to date with current practice, whilst the new Trainer will find help in the clearly laid out sequence of events in preparation for the VT year.

In providing a Vocational Training experience of equal opportunity throughout England and Wales, it has always been CVT's aim to balance the need for some degree of standardisation with the advantages of allowing Deaneries their own individuality. Your own Deanery will have provided training in preparation for taking on the task of training a young colleague in your practice. This handbook can be used as an aide-mémoire or to confirm that your plans comply with CVT guidance on a range of issues.

Help in day-to-day management of the training period is invaluable for new Trainers, whilst old hands may find some alternative ways of keeping the learning experience fresh and targeted to the VDP's needs.

Quick answers to questions on rules or guidance are often required during practice-based tutorials, or arising from a chair-side situation. It will be reassuring for many to find the answer, or reference as to where to find detailed information, simply by reaching to the bookshelf.

All good teachers undertake thorough preparation as the key to success. In this handbook you will find tools to enable you to prepare well, at the same time responding to the needs of your individual VDP. I am sure that you will find it helpful, supporting both the broad curriculum recommended by CVT and particular characteristics of your own Deanery.

Here too, you may find ideas for your personal development as a Trainer, so much encouraged in many Deaneries. The natural progression of many committed Trainers is into the crucial rôle of Adviser, and the handbook also serves the purpose of gathering together much of the information and knowledge necessary to an Adviser.

Having taken the decision to read this book you have confirmed your interest in the development of VT, and to use it will enhance your contribution to the essence of a successful training period: the relationship between Trainer and VDP.

Penelope Vasey MBE BDS DGDP(UK)
Chairman
Committee on Vocational Training for England and Wales
September 2001

COMMITTEE ON VOCATIONAL TRAINING FOR ENGLAND AND WALES

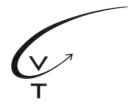

Foreword

Authorship of a book such as this, which covers the broad and comprehensive range of knowledge of the subject of vocational training in general dental practice, requires an unusual and comprehensive combination of attributes including:

- extensive experience in working as a general dental practitioner and in running a dental practice
- regular involvement in continuing professional development to ensure that clinical knowledge and ideas are up to date
- experience as a Trainer and as an Adviser in vocational training
- knowledge of the theory and experience in the application of the principles of adult education
- ability to communicate ideas and to write in an easy to read style - the subject material has to be readily absorbed by the prospective trainer or adviser with little time to spare after dental practice on a day to day basis
- tenacity and power of application to a task that requires development of new ideas and preparation of original material, and the ability to edit text to achieve a concise but comprehensive coverage of the subject.

The author Raj Rattan has demonstrated in this book that he has all these attributes. The work, which as far as I know is unique in this field, provides the necessary overall theory and also practical ideas for the new trainer in vocational dental practice, as well as useful reading for the vocational dental practitioner. In addition, it acts as a comprehensive revision text for the Trainer who already has experience, as well as for VT Advisers and Regional Advisers. It represents a text that has been carefully researched, written and edited to result in a unique distillate of knowledge and experience.

In conclusion, the abilities of the author as an experienced clinician with practice management experience, as a leader in all aspects of vocational training, as a qualified educator and as a craftsman of the written word have resulted in an invaluable and unique text of this subject area. I most strongly recommend this book to all those who are participating in, or providing, vocational training, or who are involved in any way with vocational dental practice.

Ian M Waite
Postgraduate Dental Dean
Department of Medical and Dental Education
The London Postgraduate Deanery
September 2001

Preface

Vocational training (VT) in general dental practice is a particular form of training derived from a concept known by the generic term 'on-the-job training' (OJT). OJT may be defined as training that is planned and structured, and takes place mainly in the normal working environment in which an appointed person spends time with the trainee to impart knowledge and teach new skills that have been specified in advance. It has long been recognised as the preferred method for developing practical and other workplace skills.

VT has evolved over more than 30 years into the current paradigm for in-practice learning. It relies on the principles of critical reflection, collaborative goal setting and interactive learning as well as some of the more traditional approaches to adult education. It became mandatory in October 1993 for all UK dental graduates and continues to remain under the overall control and guidance of the Committee on Vocational Training (CVT) for England and Wales.

My interest and involvement in vocational training spans almost 15 years. My first experience as a trainer led to my first presentation – on stress management. The irony is obvious now but, curiously, it wasn't at the time. Some years later I became the VT adviser for the scheme based at Whipps Cross Hospital in North London, and a few years later was appointed as a regional adviser in the same deanery.

During those 15 years, I have been a trainer and joint trainer on numerous occasions. I have enjoyed the privilege of giving over 100 presentations to vocational dental practitioners (VDPs) in all parts of the country and have enjoyed the friendship and camaraderie of my colleagues throughout this period. My work with Dental Protection Ltd as a dento-legal adviser has given me experience in handling a number of cases involving VDPs and trainers ranging from complaints, negligence cases and matters involving the General Dental Council (GDC), as well as a variety of contractual disputes.

These experiences inform this book. I was first asked by CVT to write *The Trainer's Handbook* in 1992, and then to update it two years later. This book is loosely based on that earlier text, but it has been thoroughly revised and includes a great deal of additional material. It is aimed at dentists who have an interest in vocational training and I hope it will be particularly useful to trainers, VDPs and VT advisers/Regional advisers.

In his leader, Training the trainers [*British Dental Journal* (24 July 1999)],

Peter Mossey wrote that 'General dental practitioners are primary care clinicians with experiential training in management, business and interpersonal skills ...', and went on to state that one major challenge for the profession 'will be the training of dental practitioners to become competent educators for this important role'.

I hope that this book will help to achieve that goal.

Raj Rattan
September 2001

About the author

Raj Rattan is a general dental practitioner and a Regional Adviser in vocational training in the London Deanery. He is also an adviser and consultant to a number of dental organisations. Raj is a regular contributor and columnist in the dental press and has lectured extensively in the UK and overseas on a wide range of subjects related to all aspects of general dental practice. Some of his published and lecture material has been developed into a range of teaching and training modules for use in seminar programmes run by various dental organisations including Dental Bodies Corporate and health authorities.

Acknowledgements

Dental Vocational Training would not be where it is today without the input from trainers and the dedication of the Advisers and Regional Advisers. Their collective efforts have helped to create the synergy that has formulated many of the ideas and concepts discussed in this book. It is impossible to name them all and I would risk the unfairness of omission, but I welcome this opportunity to record their commitment.

My thanks to the Committee on Vocational Training for their interest in this book and, in particular, to Penelope Vasey MBE and Sara Hall MBE for their helpful suggestions and comments before the book went to press.

I also wish to record the support and encouragement I received from Bill Allen OBE (then Chairman of CVT and Regional Adviser), during my early years in vocational training.

Like many of the readers of this book, I am a general dental practitioner and the demands of running a practice has meant that much of the work for this book has been undertaken outside surgery hours. I am indebted to my wife and children for allowing me to do this in what should have been their time.

And finally, it has been a joy to work again with the team at Radcliffe Medical Press; they have a rare gift for making their authors feel part of an extended family.

This book is dedicated to my mother.

CHAPTER 1

Trainer selection

General dental practitioners interested in becoming trainers must satisfy the Regional Trainer Selection Committee that they are eligible and suited for the role, and that their practice meets the minimum standards required of a training practice. Practitioners usually apply individually, but practitioners may also apply with a practice colleague and seek approval as joint trainers.

The Committee on Vocational Training (CVT) produces a person specification for trainers, which considers qualifications, knowledge and experience, and skills and abilities, and sets out essential and desirable criteria. These are summarised in Table 1.1.

The selection procedure comprises three parts:

1 the completion of an application form
2 a practice visit
3 an interview before a trainer selection committee.

Formal application

Application forms are available from the regional postgraduate dental dean's office and can be downloaded from the regional website. The forms do vary from region to region and may reflect regional preferences, but most seek to obtain very similar information from the applicants. Some trainers submit a CV with the form, but this is not a formal requirement. A copy of the practice visit form is available to applicants from the regional office or can be downloaded from the region's website for manual completion or electronic transmission.

The design and content of application forms are under constant review to reflect topical issues, changes in health and safety legislation and good practice guidance.

Interviews are arranged after application forms have been received and carefully considered. Some regions prefer to short-list applicants first, but this practice has been used only when large numbers of applications have been received.

Table 1.1 Trainer person specification

Attributes	Essential	Ideal
Qualifications	• A dentist who practices in the General Dental Services. • A dentist who earns the equivalent of 20% of notional Target Annual Gross Income. • A dentist in a stable relationship with his or her practice. • A principal, associate or salaried dentist who can demonstrate involvement and influence on the running of the practice and the practice policy.	• A principal with managerial responsibility who is a practice owner or an equity holder.
Knowledge and experience	• A dentist with high clinical and ethical standards. • A dentist who provides a wide range of treatment. • A dentist who can prove a commitment to postgraduate education and training by certificates or other records of attendance at recent postgraduate courses. • A dentist who understands the legal framework of general practice. • A dentist who has been in GDP practice for 4 years or more (upon initial appointment).	• A dentist under the age of 60 years (upon initial appointment). • A dentist who can prove a commitment to postgraduate education by possession of MFGDP, MGDS or other relevant qualification.
Skills and abilities	• A dentist who works as part of a team within a well-run practice. • A dentist able to cope with change, who is flexible and can handle uncertainty. • A dentist who is able to communicate effectively with patients and other team members. • A dentist who is available and accessible to patients through an efficient appointment system and other methods of access. • A dentist who is willing to re-organise own daily routine and those of the practice to take account of the presence of a VDP. • A dentist who has developed a critical faculty for self-assessment and can demonstrate this. • A dentist who can demonstrate involvement in staff training and development.	• A dentist who owns and runs a well-organised practice. • A dentist who is interested in adding knowledge to general practice or can show a commitment to continuing professional development by: – participation in peer review, clinical audit or research in general practice – recent presentations to postgraduate and continuing training courses – recent articles, reviews or letters on related topics published locally or nationally.

Reproduced with permission of CVT

In some regions, applicants may be requested to submit additional documentation with their form. Practice information leaflets, samples of staff contracts, the annual prescribing profile issued by the Dental Practice Board and evidence of compliance with a particular aspect of health and safety legislation are just some examples.

The practice visit

The practice visit is an important part of the selection procedure; its purpose is to assess the practice's suitability for vocational training. Information is recorded on a form that includes sections on the facilities available for the VDP, details of services provided and not provided, staff arrangements, compliance with good practice guidelines and aspects of health and safety legislation. Most Deaneries now ask potential trainers to complete a self-assessment practice inspection document. A copy of the form is made available to members of the selection committee prior to or at the interview stage.

In the case of new trainers, the visit is normally undertaken by two people during the working day and at a time convenient to the practitioner. In the case of existing trainers, the visit may be undertaken by one person alone, usually the VT adviser. The visit lasts approximately 1 hour, and applicants are requested to set aside this time from their clinical schedule to accommodate the visiting team. Applicants can take advantage of this time to ask any questions they may have about any aspect of VT.

It should be noted that in some regions the practice visit takes place after the selection interview. If the applicant is deemed to be a potentially suitable trainer, a practice visit is then undertaken. It therefore follows that someone who is unsuccessful at interview will not be visited. This approach is the exception rather than the rule. It occurred in those regions that were heavily over-subscribed with trainer applications and where it was therefore impractical to undertake visits for each and every applicant, given that only 12 trainers (and some reserves) would be appointed on a competitive basis. The reason for this variation is a reflection on the emphasis placed by some regions on the different parts of the application process.

Practitioners are encouraged to prepare in advance for the visit and to have the various certificates and documents that must now comply with statutory legislation ready for inspection. If there are planned changes to the practice environment, for example refurbishment or redecoration, it is always prudent to have available a summary of the proposed changes to give the visitors a good idea of what changes are in the pipeline.

The visitors will follow the regional protocol on practice visits, which normally includes:

- the completion of a practice visit questionnaire
- a review of the workload of the practice by looking at the appointment book(s)
- an examination of a random selection of record cards and radiographs
- an appraisal of the office management systems
- meeting some of the practice staff
- assessing the practice library and other educational resources available.

This last point sometimes causes concern amongst new applicants. Practitioners are expected to maintain a reasonable selection of reference books and journals, including key reference books such as the *Dental Practitioner Formulary/British National Formulary*, copies of *NHS Regulations*. Access to other educational resources such as the Internet, CD-ROMs, and videotapes would also be looked upon favourably.

In some regions, the visitors may wish to take photographs or make a video recording of the practice. This is done with the applicant's consent and total confidentiality of all records is assured.

In general terms, a practice would be considered suitable if it fulfilled certain criteria, namely that:

- the VDPs surgery is adequately equipped to permit the practice of four-handed dentistry
- sterilisation by autoclave is in routine use for items not damaged by the process
- handpieces are sterilised between patients and their supply is sufficient to permit this
- barrier protection, including gloves, masks and spectacles, is used during the treatment of patients
- correct methods of waste disposal are in place
- Ionising Radiation Regulations are observed
- the production of amalgam is by closed devices
- emergency drugs and oxygen are available
- there is evidence of compliance to good practice guidelines
- there is an out-of-hours service for the treatment of emergencies
- there is evidence of compliance with health and safety legislation
- there is adequate administrative and chairside support from a suitably experienced dental assistant.

If the practice fails to satisfy any particular requirement, the visitors will be pleased to advise on what needs to be done to remedy the situation. If, subsequently, evidence is available to confirm that shortcomings have been addressed, the application is not necessarily jeopardised and may proceed in the normal way. On occasions, and in the event of uncertainty or major changes, a follow-up visit may be recommended.

The interview

The regional trainer selection committee approves trainers and training practices. The selection committee normally includes the regional post-graduate dental dean, the regional/VT adviser, a general dental practitioner (GDP) who may be a Local Dental Committee (LDC) member, a General Dental Services Committee (GDSC) member and a representative from the FGDP.

The interview lasts approximately 30–45 minutes. The content and conduct of the interview may vary and applicants should be prepared to give their views on:

• reasons for wanting to be involved in VT
• postgraduate education activities
• items of particular interest on the application form
• previous experiences of VT
• personal strengths and weaknesses
• type of work carried out at the practice
• topics of current professional interest
• practice organisation and administration.

Notification of the outcome of the interview is by post once all the inter-views have been completed. Successful applicants are approved for one year only and reappointments are made on a competitive basis. Successful applicants are ranked in order of merit, as determined by interview. This means that a particular applicant and practice may be suitable for training purposes, but may not necessarily be selected for that particular year if they fall outside the first 12 places. In this situation, many regions will appoint reserve trainers who can step in if someone has to withdraw from the scheme for any reason. Twelve trainers are normally appointed; in addition there may be as many as three reserves.

Trainers seeking reappointment in any year following their initial appointment will be required to submit a new application in the usual way.

CHAPTER 2

The trainer's role and responsibilities

The trainer has a key role to play in the professional development of the VDP. This role, whilst not onerous, demands a continual commitment from both parties to ensure the satisfactory completion of the VT year. The responsibilities of trainers throughout the year are summarised below:

- employ a VDP in the practice under the terms of a nationally agreed contract
- prepare and conduct regular weekly tutorials for the VDP and be available to give guidance in both clinical and administrative matters by working in the same premises as the VDP for not less than three days per week
- provide the VDP with satisfactory facilities, support and relevant opportunities so that a wide range of NHS practice is experienced and, as far as is reasonably possible, the VDP is fully occupied
- assess and monitor the VDP's progress and professional development, ensuring that the professional development portfolio is maintained and kept up to date, give feedback to the VDO and liaise with the VT adviser, as necessary
- allow and require the VDP to attend the VT study course of approximately 30 days, and ensure that the VDP's holidays do not lead to absence from the study days
- acquire the skills necessary to undertake the role of trainer and to undertake training in assessment through participation in educational courses prior to the employment of a VDP in the practice and during the training period, as required
- attend trainer and assessment meetings and set time aside to be available for adviser visit(s) to the practice, as required
- advise on the final certification of the VDP's completion of VT.

The role of the trainer

The trainer takes on multiple roles during the training year. Results from surveys carried out in the late 1980s suggest that VDPs perceive the trainer to have five key roles. These are:

- mentor
- counsellor
- employer
- friend
- teacher.

All are important, but the role of teacher and mentor are particularly important in the continuum of dental education (Figure 2.1).

It is interesting to compare this list to the roles identified by general medical practitioner trainers (Caird and Ogden, 2001). These were expressed in ranked order as:

- resource
- facilitator
- mentor
- critic.

As VDPs climb the ladder of their professional experience, the dominant teaching style shifts from the passive to the interactive and finally to the self-directed. This gradual upward shift is facilitated by the people and processes shown on the right of the ladder; the role of the trainer is clearly defined in this model.

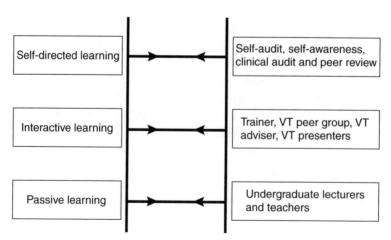

Figure 2.1 Continuum of dental education for the VDP.

Many of these roles are self-explanatory, but those of mentor and counsellor are worthy of further exploration.

Mentor

The concept of the mentor is centuries old, and we have to look to Homer's *Odyssey* to help define the original term, for it was in that classical work that Odysseus, when he went to fight in the Trojan War, entrusted his son, Telemachus, to a tutor called Mentor. In modern times, the mentor relationship has been described as 'one of the most developmentally important relationships a person can have in early adulthood'. Perhaps the greatest mentor relationship in history was that between Socrates and Plato, but there are some more recent notable examples. Academy award winner Anthony Hopkins credits his success to the influence of fellow Welshman Richard Burton, of whom he said 'He had quite an influence on my life because he got away and became an actor. And I thought – God, I'd like to do that'.

The role of the mentor has been described as:

> *a teacher to enhance the young man's skills and intellectual development. He may use his influence to promote the young man's advancement. He may be a host and a guide, welcoming the initiate into a new occupational and social world ... Through his own virtues, achievements, the way of life, the mentor may be an exemplar that the protégé can admire and seek to emulate. He may provide counsel and moral support in times of stress* (Levinson, 1979).

This quotation paints an accurate picture of the relationship that exists between trainer and VDP.

The Standing Committee on Postgraduate Medical and Dental Education (SCOPME), in its report *Supporting doctors and dentists at work: an enquiry into mentoring* described mentoring as a 'synthesis of concepts'. It defined mentoring as:

> *the process whereby an experienced, highly regarded, empathic individual (the mentor), by listening and talking in confidence, guides another individual, often but not always working in the same organisation or field (the mentee), in the development and re-examination of the mentee's own ideas, learning, personal and professional development ...* (SCOPME, 1998).

Studies involving mentoring relationships have identified highly valued aspects of the relationship (Bova and Phillips, 1981). These were shown to be:

• communication skills
• survival within the system
• skills of their profession
• respect and understanding of people
• setting high standards
• how to be a good listener
• leadership qualities
• what it means to be professional
• how to manage a team.

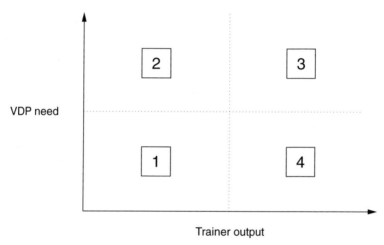

Figure 2.2   Matching resources to need.

The extent to which the relationship is allowed to flourish within VT is largely dependent on the circumstances of situations. These can be summarised in a simple matrix comprising four quadrants (Figure 2.2).

The first quadrant reflects low levels of need and low levels of input; the input will be infrequent and often spontaneous. In the second quadrant, the need may be high but the resources are limited and this is where others may need to become involved to provide the necessary input to meet the VDP's expectation. A good example would be the involvement of both trainers in a joint trainer relationship. The third quadrant is possibly the most productive; high demand matches ample resources and this category probably represents the best and most productive relationships. In quadrant 4, the trainer can easily meet the requirements and the surplus resources may be redirected to helping others within the practice.

Trainers should consider adopting the ABC model of mentoring:

A achieve a relationship
B boil the problem down: formative and supportive roles
C challenge the VDP to change or cope.

(Sanders, 1998)

Another facet of mentoring is sometimes described as 'peer mentoring'. A number of universities in the USA now use the principle that is based on the observation that learners perform better if they are comfortable with their environment and circumstances. Fellow members of the VT scheme may act as peer mentors, as may other dentists within the practice who may have participated in a previous scheme. The role of the peer mentor is therefore slightly different from that of the trainer.

Counsellor

Counselling is a process that helps individuals to:

- identify problems
- analyse feelings
- create problem-solving pathways
- accept the inevitable.

It should always take place on a confidential basis and in an environment free from interruptions and distractions. The process may involve a combination of the following:

- helping the VDP in the decision-making process
- giving advice
- discussing a problem of which the VDP may not be aware (e.g. a patient complaint)
- helping to alter perceptions
- providing moral support in difficult times.

Two counselling techniques are widely recognised. These are known as non-directive and directive counselling, the characteristics of which are summarised overleaf.

Non-directive counselling
The features of non-directive counselling are:

- counsellee defines the problem
- both parties propose solutions
- implement solution with which both parties agree.

Directive counselling
The features of directive counselling are:

- counsellor is dominant
- both parties define problem
- counsellor proposes solution.

Whatever methods are used, they have many things in common. In general terms, the ten key factors in successful counselling are:

1 give the VDP support and reassurance
2 maintain a good relationship with the VDP
3 listen to the VDP without being judgemental
4 try to give them an explanation of what has happened
5 if asked, suggest a range of solutions
6 give the VDP an opportunity to express their emotions freely
7 boost their confidence in the context of your interaction
8 encourage the adoption of empowering beliefs and attitudes
9 give them a sense of a positive outcome and hope
10 maintain the relationship after the interaction.

The characteristics of the roles of friend, teacher and employer will already be familiar and the reader is referred to other sections of this book for a more detailed review of what is expected of trainers in their role as teachers.

CHAPTER 3

Selecting your VDP

Trainers are responsible for VDP recruitment. In some parts of the country, particularly in and around big cities, the competition for training places is intense and it is not uncommon for training practices to receive up to 50 or 60 applications, and sometimes more. In contrast, practices in more remote areas may have some difficulty in attracting a reasonable number of applicants.

Once approved, the local postgraduate office publishes an official list of approved practices. Some regions produce paper lists but all now publish the information on their website. Trainers will be asked to supply a brief synopsis of their practice and this information will be included in the list.

Eligibility

In order for a dentist to be eligible to undertake vocational training, he or she must possess a qualification registrable with the General Dental Council. Eligibility does not of course guarantee entry onto a VT scheme because the places are limited and subject to open competition. In addition, the Department of Health will not fund the training of dentists who plan to leave the UK immediately after completing the course or who are not eligible to remain here for 12 months or more at the start of their VT. Anyone who may not be publicly funded should undertake VT only within the Training and Work Experience Scheme (TWES). A trainer would have to apply for a work permit under TWES and the potential VDP would need to be funded from a source other than the NHS.

The eligibility criteria to undertake VT are summarised in Figure 3.1.

Trainers should note that it is now a criminal offence to employ anyone aged 16 or over who is not legally entitled to live and work in the UK. A trainer can avoid committing this offence (under Section 8 of the Asylum and Immigration Act 1996) by building simple and straightforward checks into the normal recruitment process. Records should be kept to provide a statutory defence in case of prosecution. To avoid separate prosecution under the Race Relations Act 1976 all applicants for a post at

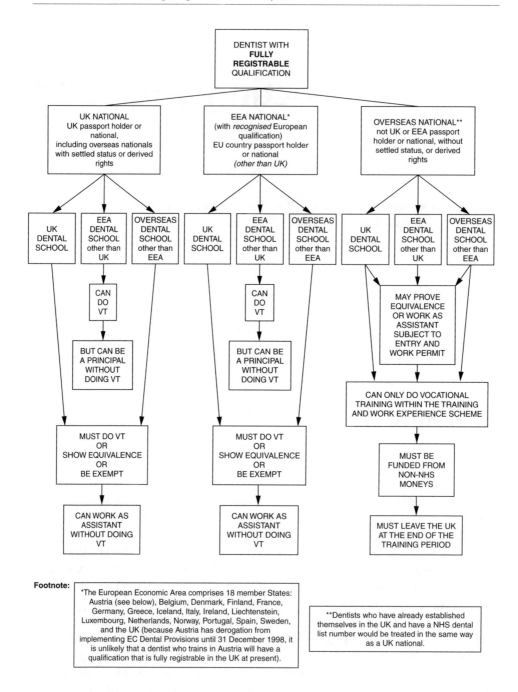

Figure 3.1 Eligibility of dentists to undertake VT and work in NHS general dental practice (reproduced with permission of CVT).

the practice must be treated in the same non-discriminatory way. As employees, VDPs must be treated equally.

Business and commercial arrangements

With effect from 1 October 2000, the skills' threshold for the business and commercial arrangements changed. The changes now enable some applications that were considered under TWES to be considered for a full work permit, under the business and commercial arrangements.

Of the four optional criteria that an applicant must have in order to meet the skills' criteria and obtain a work permit under the arrangements, one is directly applicable to dental vocational training – that an overseas national must have a UK degree level qualification.

Employers should apply under the arrangements using Form WP1 and WP1 Notes of Guidance. The application would need to meet the full criteria of the arrangements including a resident search. Further details can be found in the Notes of Guidance.

Trainers can also find useful information such as the Code of Practice on the Immigration and Asylum Act 1999 on the Employers' Information section of the Immigration and Nationality Directorate's website: www.ind.homeoffice.gov.uk .

Advertising the post

It is perhaps a useful reminder for new trainers, and particularly those in more remote areas, that the advertisement should be designed to appeal to the recent graduate. As well as including an outline of the facilities available within the practice it is also a good idea to mention:

- accommodation availability
- public transport access
- leisure facilities
- opportunities for social interaction
- other unique features of the location and environment
- previous experience of VT.

It is surprising how many VDPs target practices for reasons other than internal facilities, so maximum advantage should be taken of any unique features.

When writing the practice description, remember the trusted advertising acronym AIDA:

A ttention
I nterest
D esire
A ction.

A description that gets the readers *attention* will create *interest* and then a *desire* for positive *action*.

If the practice has a current VDP, some trainers have felt it an advantage to include a recommendation (where appropriate!) from that person, and offer interviewees an opportunity to discuss the post with the incumbent VDP on an informal basis.

Some training practices choose to advertise in the dental press, or will contact dental schools directly and advise them of the vacancy. This happens less often now that mandatory VT is in place and there is a demand for places.

The lists of training practices are published on the Deanery website, which potential VDPs can access directly or via the CVT website. Some Deaneries include detailed practice descriptions and photographs, whereas others provide links to a practice's own website, where available.

The selection process

Trainers should decide how they want potential applicants to make first contact with the practice.

The vast majority of trainers invite applications by CV. It is increasingly common for trainers to receive telephone calls or letters of inquiry from final year students before the official lists have been published because some students make inquiries of current VDPs and will make speculative submissions to them. The majority of trainers prefer to wait until lists have been formally published and the majority of applications have been received before they commence the short-listing.

In many cases, the first part of the selection procedure is to review the CV of applicants. It is very difficult to make objective decisions from CVs alone. Many CVs are very similar and the widespread use of word processors and CV templates means that many arrive in similar formats. It is up to the individual trainer how much emphasis they wish to place on each section of the CV. Some prefer graduates with a track record of academic excellence whilst others will focus on their experience of 'hands-on' dentistry. Some prefer graduates from particular undergraduate schools, whilst others chose to ignore these factors and focus on applicants' hobbies and social interests.

Trainers should be aware of two factors that will affect how the selection process is carried out. First, it should be recognised that not all train-ing practices receive the same number of applications. As has been stated earlier, practices in and around big cities tend to attract more applica-tions. The selection process for this group of trainers will be more involved. It is important that the selection process is conducted in an orderly and equitable way. All applications should be treated in the same way and the process should follow established guidelines.

• Set a closing date for applications.
• Advise all potential applicants of that date.
• Review all the CVs and then prepare a short-list.
• Organise one or more interviews for the short-listed applicants.

Some training practices may receive only a handful of applications and may prefer to short-list all applicants and interview each in turn.

Second, many graduates will make multiple applications to training practices. It is very likely that the outstanding cohort of applicants will be identified by a number of trainers who have interviewed them. The corol-lary is that a number of applicants from this group will receive multiple offers of employment. They will then be in the enviable position of being able to choose their trainer(s) and/or training practice. It is important to recognise that inefficient selection processes can disadvantage the inex-perienced trainer in particular because the pool of suitable candidates will have been depleted by those who have been quick off the mark in their selection.

The interview

A great deal has been written about interview techniques and the unreli-ability of the process is well documented and borne out by the practical experience of many trainers. The purpose of the interview should be to:

• confirm factual details
• gain an insight into an applicant's personality
• assess personal life experience
• assess professional experience
• provide practice information
• conduct a tour of the practice
• invite questions.

The first stage of the selection procedure should be to think about the sort of person who would be suitable for the practice, taking into consideration

their abilities and qualifications. It can be useful to prepare a person specification with 'essential' and 'desirable' attributes in much the same way as
a person specification exists for trainers (*see* Table 1.1). A version of this
should be used for criterion-based short-listing. Include criteria that relate
to the organisation and management of the practice itself. For example, it
may be important that the VDP demonstrates a willingness to work late on
a particular day when there is an evening surgery. It will not be possible to
assess some of these things from the CV alone and the specification for
short-listing should include only those items that can be easily assessed
from the CV.

The National Institute of Industrial Psychology has conducted much
interesting research into interview techniques and the assessment of
applicants. Its research suggests that candidates should be assessed
under six broad headings. These are:

- attainments
- general intelligence
- special aptitude
- interests
- disposition
- circumstances.

Attainments are special skills and abilities normally gained as a result of
much effort over a prolonged period of time. These can be assessed from
the candidate's CV.

The objective measurement of general intelligence and special aptitudes is difficult at interview unless the candidate has exceptional
qualities that come to light during the course of the interview. As university graduates and professionals, all have proven abilities. Prizes, awards
and references often give a valuable insight into a candidate's special
aptitudes.

Outline information about professional and personal interests and
hobbies are normally indicated on the CV. Candidates are usually only
too pleased to elaborate on their hobbies and interests and should be
given an opportunity to do so.

Disposition refers to the way someone tends to behave and feel and
this will become evident during the interview.

A candidate's personal circumstances including where they live, ease of
travel to the practice and motivation will all have a bearing on the
outcome of the interview.

Quite often, interviews in the practice take place with more than one
interviewer. Each interviewer should receive an assessment form and the
results should be analysed at the conclusion of the interview. There are

numerous examples of interview record forms and a simple format is shown in Box 3.1. Note that a numerical scoring system is not universally accepted. Some people recommend the use of words and phrases such as 'adequate', 'satisfactory', 'exemplary', which can be underlined to indicate the interviewer's perception of the applicant. If a numerical scoring system is used, it is helpful to keep to an even number to prevent interviewers scoring a central average.

Interview technique

Interview skills, like many management techniques, are acquired skills. Natural aptitude helps but many dentists have had to learn the hard way. There may not be a substitute for experience, but there are some general principles that will facilitate the process and may help to make the outcome more predictable. Many studies indicate that the interview is a very poor method of predicting performance. It retains its popularity

---

Box 3.1 Interview assessment form

QUALITIES			RATING			

Personal

Interpersonal skills	1	2	3	4	5	6
Communication skills	1	2	3	4	5	6
Appearance						
Attitude	1	2	3	4	5	6

Professional

Practice	1	2	3	4	5	6
Special interests	1	2	3	4	5	6
Education	1	2	3	4	5	6
Ambition	1	2	3	4	5	6
Commitment to practice	1	2	3	4	5	6
Understanding of VT	1	2	3	4	5	6

General comments

....

....

....

....

largely because of administrative convenience and a lack of equivalent assessment methods.

The interview is one of the most commonly used assessment tools. Many trainers conduct interviews with a view to trying to predict the likely future performance of the candidate. Despite its widespread use, the concept of *predictive validity* has been challenged and questioned by psychologists for many years. In some studies the predictive validity co-efficient has been as low as 0.16 (measured on a scale of 0–1), which does rather suggest that the interview is perhaps not the most reliable tool.

If predictive validity is an important issue, then other assessment tools, such as activity tests and on-the-job tasks must be used. It is not practical to undertake this and so the interview remains the cornerstone of the selection process. Some trainers will however prepare a list of typical practice scenarios, some clinical and some not, and ask the candidates to give their views on how they would deal with the situations presented in the scenarios.

There are several ways of improving the effectiveness of interviews:

Prepare a clear job specification
This will help you formulate objectives for the position and will provide a reference point for the candidate. Although a nationally agreed trainer–VDP contract is in place, the job description should reflect the requirements of the post, that are specific to the individual practice, but should not conflict with the overall aims and objectives of vocational training.

Consult with practice colleagues
Many trainers involve members of the dental team in recognition of the fact that it is often the strength of the interpersonal relationships, which underpins the successful practice. VDPs are more likely to be embraced by all members of the team if they have been represented during the selection process.

Prepare a structure to the interview
One way of improving the reliability of interviews is to reduce the number of variables. Giving the interview some structure and format can do this. A lack of structure usually results in the interview being little more than a 'conversation' between the two parties and the benefit of the information gained is limited. The interview should be a formal affair conducted in an orderly fashion.

Many VDPs have reported their experience of the interview process and it has been the view of a sizeable number that many interviews lacked organisation and structure. Many complained that their time had been wasted and that the interview was nothing more than a '10-minute' chat, frequently slotted in between patients or crammed into the lunch hour alongside other non-clinical commitments.

The advantages of a structured interview have been demonstrated in many large organisations. Many interviews follow a pattern that focuses on work experience, education, social contacts, own beliefs and attitudes and future plans – topics that largely repeat the information in the candidate's CV. Research reinforces the importance of structure over content and it has been shown that the predictive validity rating in a structured interview is double that of an unstructured process.

It can be useful to devise a standard procedure, which could include a tour of the practice, a written summary of the job, an application form to complete and an introduction to the interviewer(s). If you intend to take notes, tell the candidates first so that they are not distracted during the interview. Keep the notes brief at this stage because it can be off-putting for young and inexperienced candidates. More detailed comments can always be jotted down at the end of the interview.

Picture the ideal candidate

This has already been discussed briefly. It is a useful technique in which the interviewer writes down the desirable characteristics of the ideal candidate and then measures the applicants against them. It is essential that you know what sort of person you are looking for. Adhering to the old adage 'I don't know what I want, but I'll know when I find it' is at best a cavalier approach to selection and reminiscent of the *laissez-faire* school of management.

Types of questions

A range and variety of questions can provide trainers with a great deal of information about potential VDPs. Ask open questions as much as possible. Open questions encourage applicants to give their views and are a good way of teasing out attitudes. A question like *What is your approach to patient care?* will give far more information about a candidate's views and attitudes than a question that, for example, sets out the practice policy on patient care and simply asks *Do you agree with that?* The latter is an example of a leading question and an interviewee is hardly likely to disagree with your practice policy.

A double question is another good route of enquiry. It is two questions in one. For example, *What are your weaknesses in clinical dentistry and how do you think you will address these?*

Examples of open interview questions are given in Box 3.2.

Box 3.2 Sample questions

- Tell me about an occasion where you felt you had to use your initiative.
- Give me an example of an occasion where you exceeded your own expectations.
- I see from your CV that you were involved with the Student's Association. How do you rate that experience?
- Where do you see yourself in five years?
- When was the last time you were involved in a conflict situation and how did you deal with it?
- In your opinion what makes a good dentist?
- Now tell me what you think makes a great dentist.
- Who do you think is responsible for your professional development this year?
- What are your strengths and weaknesses?
- In what ways do you think vocational training differs from undergraduate training?
- How will you know if you have been successful this year?
- What are the current hot topics in dentistry?

Avoid discriminatory questions such as *How do you feel about working in a practice where all the other dentists are male*? Not only is this a leading question, but there are also equal opportunity considerations to bear in mind. It is better to avoid questions on religion, colour, race, national origin, marital status, sex, childcare and family matters.

It has been said that the best guide to future performance of a candidate is past behaviour. Behavioural questions such as *How will you ensure that you make the most of the training opportunities at this practice?* can provide some interesting clues as to the candidate's likely future performance.

Bias

One reason that interviews are not wholly reliable is to do with bias. The most common types of bias are age, sex, race, attitude, appearance, non-verbal behavioural cues and the physical setting of the interview. Another important and often omitted facet of bias relates to market conditions at the time. Receiving fewer applications than anticipated can lead to the selection of a less than ideal candidate because of lack of choice.

Impression management is the term used to indicate certain forms of bias. There are some interesting observations in this respect. For example, it has been found that females who dress in more masculine clothes stand a better chance of being selected for management positions than those who appear more feminine. Perfumed applicants, both male and female, are more likely to rate highly with female interviewers than with male interviewers.

Three other frequently occurring phenomena are:

* stereotyping
* the halo effect
* central tendency.

Stereotyping occurs when an individual forms a fixed opinion of someone that leads to the assumption that he or she will behave in a particular way.

The halo effect occurs when the interviewer recognises one particular characteristic in the applicant and allows it to bias the remainder of the interview. For example, if an applicant for a practice manager's job is attractively attired, the interviewer may be so impressed with the candidate's dress that he or she assumes the applicant will be competent in a managerial capacity. It can work in reverse. If, for example, an applicant attends for interview dressed inappropriately it may create a poor impression, tarnishing the interviewer's perception of the candidate's attributes (which may have been more than satisfactory).

Central tendency occurs when an interviewer averages everything rather than giving high or low ratings, which require more justification. The interview rating scale suggested in Box 3.1 uses a six-point assessment thus preventing the interviewer awarding a central average.

To summarise, the key features of good interview technique are:

* to prepare in advance
* to put the candidate at ease
* to read and absorb the information on the candidate's application
* to ask open questions and maintain a logical sequence
* to encourage the candidate to do most of the talking
* to not let personal prejudice interfere with the conduct of the interview
* to maintain a polite and courteous manner throughout
* to provide the candidate with accurate information about the training position.

It is important to be consistent with each candidate in order to ensure that comparisons are valid.

Interview experiences

It is interesting to review the responses to questionnaires that were sent to trainers and VDPs to seek their views on the interview process. The study highlighted some important concerns about the process, many of which have been discussed in this text (British Dental Journal, 1997). The responses from trainers are shown in Table 3.1.

Table 3.1 Trainers' responses

		Yes n (%)	No n (%)
1	Have you been a trainer before?	53 (74)	19 (26)
2	Did you receive sufficient help from either a dental school or CVT in helping to select candidates to interview?	47 (65)	24 (33)
3	Did you think a CV was important in choosing a potential VDP trainee?	64 (89)	8 (11)
4	Did you seek references on all candidates before interviewing?	8 (11)	64 (89)
5	Did you seek references from the dental school before appointing the VDP?	42 (58)	29 (40)
6	Did you ring or ask advice about a potential VDP at their dental school before appointing them?	30 (42)	41 (57)
7	Did you inform unsuccessful candidates whom you had interviewed that the post had been filled?	62 (86)	10 (14)
8	Were the VDPs generally well prepared for the interview?	66 (92)	6 (8)
9	Did you get any impression that any VDPs were influenced by your gender or race?	27 (37)	44 (61)
10	Did the place of qualification or dental school influence your decision on appointing the VDP?	20 (28)	50 (69)
11	Are you looking forward to the peer interaction between trainers?	69 (96)	3 (4)

Seventy-one per cent of trainers relied on 'intuitive judgement' in selecting their VDP, citing 'personality' as their main reason for appointing the successful applicant, and 19% said their decision was based on the 'professional manner' of the applicant.

Four out of five VDPs felt that trainers were biased in the selection process and identified genderism or racism as possible causes of that bias.

The authors of the study noted that 'trainers should take care when interviewing candidates not to give the wrong impression' in view of 'the potential for litigation (that) exists when competition for places in the right location is so intense'.

The authors recommend a 'careful and consistent approach' to the selection process to avoid any irregularities.

Selection tests

Four types of selection tests are widely used to assess candidates. These are:

1 personality tests
2 achievement tests
3 aptitude tests
4 intelligence tests.

Whilst these are not widely used by trainers, some believe that personality tests in particular have an important role to play in the selection process. Results can be difficult to analyse, particularly with candidates who know what the test is trying to achieve and whose answers therefore tend to reflect what is expected.

As an example, The Work Attitude Scale is often used to screen individuals for basic-skill mix posts, which could include clerical work, retailing and sales and marketing. The questionnaire comprises 44 questions that require simply yes/no answers. This type of questionnaire does not purport to assess skills, but aims to develop a profile of an applicant in terms of adaptability, ability to work within a team, attitude to work etc. In this way, the scale measures:

• service orientation – a people/environment focus
• task focus – application based
• work approach.

A detailed discussion of these methods is beyond the scope of this book, but the reader is referred to specialist texts on the subject – *see* Aitken (1996).

The final decision

At the end of the interview, remember to indicate to the interviewee when a decision is likely, and how they will be notified. Ensure that the candidate has made adequate provision to get home safely, particularly if interviews are taking place late in the day. Some trainers will also consider reimbursing travel expenses.

It is worth noting that the majority of potential VDPs applying for training positions will do so in the months leading up to their final professional examinations and it is a very stressful time for them. Many will be travelling long distances and in some cases will need to sacrifice the entire day to fulfil their interview commitment. Trainers should be sympathetic to this and ensure that the interview arrangements are organised and conducted in a way that is considerate to the interviewee's circumstances.

It is always a good idea to telephone the successful candidate and invite him or her to accept the position. The offer should be confirmed in writing immediately and the VDP should be asked to sign a letter of intent to employ and be employed, which is available from the deanery. It should be noted that final year students, who attend for interview and accept the position, cannot sign the contract because they are not qualified dentists. That is the purpose of the letter of intent. Those who are already qualified can sign the contract in the normal way.

As a matter of professional courtesy, unsuccessful candidates should also be informed.

Preventing illegal working within VT

It is a criminal offence to employ anyone aged 16 or over, who is not legally entitled to live and work in the United Kingdom. Trainers can avoid committing this offence (under section 8 of the Asylum and Immigration Act 1996) by building simple checks into the recruitment process. It is also important to keep records to provide a statutory defence in case of prosecution.

Trainers may refer to the Home Office booklet on the subject for further guidance.

CHAPTER 4

The early weeks

The early weeks in general practice have a significant effect on both the pace and the quality of the VDP's professional development. A planned and well-balanced start can contribute much in the way of self-confidence and assurance for both the trainer and the VDP. In stark contrast, the VDP who is thrown in at the deep end on the first day with all but the faintest idea on practice procedures will suffer the consequences of inadequate preparation. It is all too easy to destroy self-esteem and shatter confidences during the early weeks.

Getting started

The completion of a number of formal procedures is necessary before the VDP can start work. Trainers should confirm that the VDP has:

• registered his or her basic dental qualification with the GDC
• current membership with an indemnity provider.

Trainers should request to see evidence of this before the contract is signed. The status of registration must be full and not temporary registration. A dentist whose basic dental degree is only eligible for temporary registration may not practise in the UK except in approved hospital posts, and is not eligible to work in general dental practice.

With these fundamentals in place, trainers and the VDP will need to complete a variety of paperwork involving the postgraduate dental dean's office, the health authority (HA), the DPB and the Inland Revenue. It is advisable to complete the necessary paperwork as soon as possible after its receipt to ensure that there is no delay to the anticipated start date. Trainers must avoid the situation where the VDP is unnecessarily delayed from starting work because of outstanding paperwork.

The various forms that need to be completed, where they originate from and to whom they should be sent on completion are summarised in Table 4.1. If there is any problem with these, the scheme organisers or the staff of the postgraduate dental dean's office will be pleased to help.

In addition to these, special attention is drawn to the nationally agreed trainer–VDP contract, copies of which are available from the local Deanery and can be downloaded from the CVT website. Trainers are advised to read this through with their VDP and to refer to the guidance notes to

Table 4.1 Checklist for getting started

Organisation	Forms	Action	Notes
The local deanery	1 Letter of approval 2 'Confirmation of approval' certificate (three copies)	Trainer to sign part B of 'Confirmation of approval' certificate	Send one copy back to the dean's office, send one copy to the HA and retain one copy for reference.
	3 Trainer–VDP contract	Sign all copies	Send one copy to the dean's office, with one copy retained by both trainer and VDP.
The health authority (HA)	1 'Starter pack' 2 FP 81 form 3 DSP 1 form	1 Fill forms in 'Starter pack' 2 Trainers and VDPs to sign 3 Complete DSP 1	The FP81 will give the HA information to complete form DSP 3, a copy of which is sent to the DPB. Send form DSP 1 to the DPB in SAE provided. This advises the DPB about banking arrangements for the schedule fees.
The DPB	DPB paperwork is normally included with the 'Starter pack' from the HA	Return DSP 1 to DPB	The DPB will pay the training grant and reimburse the trainee's salary on the next available schedule. This arrangement remains in force for the training year unless the DPB is advised of any change of circumstances.
The Inland Revenue	Obtain VDP's P45, if they have one. If not, trainer completes P46 and trainee completes P15	Send P45, or P46/P15 to tax office	On receipt of P46/P15, the tax office will issue a P45 with the correct tax code.
The practice	1 Sign trainer/VDP contract 2 Complete above mentioned paperwork	1 Pay the VDP promptly 2 Provide an itemised payslip	Payment should be made on the agreed date as entered in the trainer/VDP contract.

clarify any ambiguities. One copy of this contract is retained by each of the parties, and the third copy must be returned to the deanery. The process requirements are summarised below:

- sign contract
- inform HA and submit documentation to confirm appointment
- complete starter pack
- send DSP 1 to DPB
- await contract number
- inform Inland Revenue
- pay promptly
- check reimbursement on schedule.

Induction programme

VDPs may experience feelings of uncertainty, insecurity and occasionally inadequacy when they first start in general dental practice and the main purpose of induction is to facilitate their integration with the profession and the practice. It is a process with which most trainers will be familiar because it should take place whenever a new employee joins the practice. In the case of the VDP, some aspects will need special attention because for many working as part of a team will be a new experience.

Trainers are encouraged to introduce their VDP as a professional colleague to staff and patients in order to avoid any misunderstanding of their status. The word 'trainee' was used for many years in VT but has now been superseded by 'vocational dental practitioner' for that very reason.

An example of a practice induction programme is shown in Box 4.1. It has been divided into sections for convenience. It should be noted that some aspects of induction may take place weeks after the commencement of the year and opportunities for others, like meeting financial advisers, may not necessarily arise. Such meetings are part of modern practice and the VDP should not be excluded from them. If confidential issues are under discussion, introductions can be postponed until these matters have been dealt with.

The amount of information that the VDP is expected to assimilate in the early weeks of practice is staggering. The presentation of this information can be made more interesting by:

- involving other members of the dental team
- discussing the culture and values of the practice
- providing written information for the VDP to review in their own time
- using a variety of resources.

Box 4.1 VDP induction checklist

Professional

- the HA
- the LDC
- the BDA
- FGDP
- local practitioners
- specialist practitioners

Practice based

- history
- structure
- facilities
- layout
- location of services
- referral protocols
- laboratories
- health and safety
- disposal of clinical waste
- emergency drugs
- record keeping
- management systems
- clinical governance
- practice protocols
- practice policies
- complaints procedure

VT surgery based

- air, water and power supply
- chair functions
- delivery unit functions
- handpiece function
- operating light functions and maintenance
- x-ray set function and usage
- laboratories
- equipment care and maintenance
- fault reporting
- start up and shut down procedures
- consumables and stock control system

People based

- introduction to team members
- roles and responsibilities
- management structure
- secondary care providers
- local personalities
- laboratory technicians
- maintenance engineers
- dental representatives
- accountants
- financial advisers
- bank managers
- HA dental advisers
- neighbours
- contractors

Induction should be seen as part of a continuous process that starts at the recruitment stage and continues throughout the first few weeks of the training year. Information is best provided in discrete segments interspersed with other work. This helps its understanding and acceptance.

There is sometimes a tendency to cut short the induction programme in order to 'get on with the real work of treating patients'. The dangers of this are:

- poor integration into the team
- low morale
- reduced productivity
- under-performance
- poor motivation
- equipment malfunction.

These factors can combine to lower the impact of the entire training programme and can have serious consequences on the financial viability of the VDP as far as the business of dentistry is concerned.

Planning the first week

Trainers should plan their first week in consultation with the VDP. This establishes the important precedent of joint preparation and bodes well for the remainder of the training year.

A sample timetable for the first week is shown in Table 4.2. Trainers should allow spaces in their own appointment book to help with induction training and to spend time with the VDPs, as is indicated in the timetable. Early guidance and a positive start will pay dividends later.

When planning the first week, do remember that VDPs will require more time with their patients for consultation appointments and for treatment sessions than trainers may normally allow. Make sure that support staff are aware of this and are prepared for it.

Time management skills are important in general practice and VDPs should be aware of the need for efficient practising methods. Emphasis on time management in the early stages of training is considered inappropriate, but it should be noted that efficiency is not the same as working quickly!

Remember to avoid overload in the early weeks by controlling the flow of patients and the time reserved in the appointment book. The number of patients seen in any one day in the first week will depend on what procedures have been booked in and how much time has been allowed for them. In one recent survey of practice activity levels, the average number

Table 4.2 Sample work schedule for the first week

Monday	Tuesday	Wednesday	Thursday	Friday	Notes
9.00–9.15 Welcome and introductions	**9.00–10.00** Outline practice procedures Cover more areas from induction checklist	**9.00–1.00** Treatment of patients	**9.00–1.00** Patient list	**STUDY DAY COURSE** **If no study course then repeat the format of previous days and extend induction training to include outstanding items**	The suggested timetable may be varied to suit the practice and the VDP. Some VDPs may already have experience of general practice because they may have worked as assistants. Their needs in the early part of the year will relate more to practice procedures and systems rather than aspects of working within the NHS.
9.15–10.00 Check surgery layout and function – use induction checklist	**10.00–12.30** Treatment session	**1.00–2.00** Lunch with team members	**1.00–2.00** Lunch with trainer		Some of the time allocated for induction may form part of the tutorial requirement. Any time spent over and above the base requirement should be logged and records maintained about what aspects were discussed during the session(s).
10.00–11.00 NHS forms, FP17, FPDC The SDR Record keeping Use of prescriptions	**12.30–2.00** Extended lunch Review morning session Problem solving	**2.00–5.00** Treatment session	**2.00–4.00** Treatment session		The timetable is not prescriptive, but does highlight the importance of making time available for the VDP in the first week.
11.00–12.30 Allow VDP to sit in trainer's surgery Demonstrate patient management style Involve VDP in process of treatment planning, consent and record keeping	**2.00–3.00** Tutorial on record keeping, professional development portfolio, correspondence and referral policy	**5.00–5.30** Review of the day Problem solving	**4.00–5.30** Review of the week Completion of induction Look ahead to first study day		
12.30–2.00 Extended lunch break with trainer Review afternoon daylist for VDP	**3.00–5.00** Treatment session				
2.00–5.00 VDP treatment session Book lightly	**5.00–5.30** Review of afternoon and plan ahead				
5.00–5.30 Review of afternoon Problem solving Look ahead to next day					

of patients seen per day in the first week of practice was ten. The range on any given day during the first week was between four and 16.

The key points to bear in mind are:

- avoid overload
- allow time for orientation revision
- provide an experienced dental assistant
- allow time to review the day's activities
- look ahead to the next day's appointment schedule
- go through patient records with the VDP before the day/session
- be prepared to give help on demand
- provide ample and adequate ancillary support
- be aware of early problems
- monitor VDP's time management skills
- plan your own working week to accommodate the VDP's wish for assessment if needed.

The completion of a first week in practice is a milestone for the VDP, and the first impressions of practice will have a lasting impact on their perception of general practice for several months to come.

Training needs analysis (TNA)

TNA is a process of comprehensive analysis and identification on which decisions can be made on the priorities, structure, content and process of training in the general dental practice. It is an ongoing process to steer the VDP towards more effective and efficient clinical practice, which in turn will reflect on practice performance.

There are a number of ways in which TNA can take place during the early weeks. These include:

- SWOT analysis
- performance analysis
- task analysis
- competency studies
- training needs survey
- appraisal.

The SWOT analysis

A SWOT analysis should be carried out soon after the VDP has been appointed, and, ideally, one week before the VDP is due to start work.

This gives the trainer time to plan the early part of the in-practice training schedule.

The analysis is a crude form of needs assessment at the start of the training year. Accurately identifying the VDP's early needs provides a useful frame of reference within which both the trainer and VDP can work to develop the most appropriate training programme.

SWOT is an acronym for:

- strengths
- weaknesses
- opportunities
- threats.

Strengths
The majority of VDPs list their current knowledge base as their greatest strength. Trainers are obliged to help them build on this foundation during the training year.

Weaknesses
The most common weaknesses relate to lack of clinical experience and the anxieties and fears associated with the launch of a new career.

Opportunities
The vocational training year is looked upon by many VDPs as a year of opportunity during which they expect to develop their knowledge and learn new and practical skills.

Threats
VDPs may feel threatened by what they perceive to be the stress of general practice. It is the responsibility of the trainers to ensure that undue pressure is not placed on their VDPs during this crucial period in their career.

When this analysis is complete, trainers and VDPs can begin to plan the early weeks in practice. Trainers are encouraged to work closely with the VDP and firmly establish their mutual responsibilities in planning the VDP's professional development. It is very difficult to develop this rapport later in the year if earlier opportunities have been ignored. The old adage, that advises 'to start as you mean to continue', is very apt in this relationship.

A group of VDPs was asked a series of questions relating to the trainer's input in vocational training. The answers are summarised in Box 4.2.

Box 4.2 Summary of responses from VDPs to these questions

1 INITIAL WORRIES

When you first joined your practice, what were your main concerns and anxieties?

Answers:
- working quickly enough; running on time
- not getting on with the staff; not getting on with my nurse
- the principal being fair
- not getting assistance when I need it
- my trainer's impression of my work
- the nurse's impression of my work
- dealing with difficult patients
- working in the hard, real world
- starting drilling again after a two months' break
- whether I would be able to remember how to practice dentistry after more than two years
- my first full-time job
- whether I would cope with everything, forms, dentistry, etc.
- whether it was financially worthwhile doing vocational training
- whether I would have been better off financially and educationally if I had done an associateship.

2 ON ARRIVAL

What did your trainer do that was initially most useful, helpful or supportive?

Answers:
- helped in every aspect of getting used to a new job and I was not put under any pressure at all
- lent me £500 to tide me over; paid on account until wages came through
- let me watch other associates at work for one hour per day in first week
- introduced me to the associate I have found to be most approachable throughout the year and who I turn to first

- stressed that I could work at my own pace and not to rush; told me that booking times were at my own discretion; allowed me time to treat each patient
- took me to the sports club and his or her house for meals
- introduced me to staff
- explained the NHS regulations
- gave me his or her nurse
- allowed me to spend my first day in the practice without booking patients
- booked many administration tutorials
- told me that he or she was not going to be looking over my shoulder all the time
- left me alone and only offered help when requested.

What did your trainer do that was unhelpful, or did not do that would have been helpful?

Answers:
- did not talk to me before I started
- explained to a patient that to become a dentist took six years
- was initially quite sarcastic about some of the things that I was doing, which made me even less likely to ask for help
- did not help me to find accommodation
- did not introduce me to people in the practice – it was a case of introduce yourself.

3 THE FIRST MONTH

What did your trainer do that was most useful, helpful or supportive over the first month?

Answers:
- changed my unrealistic expectations of practice by explaining the ins and outs of treatment planning and NHS regulations; helped with treatment planning
- case discussions; regular tutorials to discuss problems
- got me out of sticky situations a few times
- went through the basics of diagnosis
- kept a low profile

- allowed time to be taken; I was under no time pressure and allowed to build up at my own pace
- gave help on demand
- gave me more qualified nurses to work with
- trained new nurse.

4 THE NEXT FIVE MONTHS

What has your trainer done that has helped you most over the next five months?

Answers:
- speeded me up and prepared me for associateship
- got me out of trouble a few times
- left me alone to get on with things
- offered reassurance
- offered support
- always been happy to help out.

What has your trainer done that has been least helpful, or has not done that would have been helpful?

Answers:
- he did not really have the time during the day to discuss cases chairside, which I would have liked to do, e.g. ortho cases, complex treatment plans etc.; tended to be less available for help
- put pressure on appointment book
- did not fulful obligations with tutorials
- sat me down and gave me tutorials on things I already knew about and things that are out of date
- referred less desirable patients to me that he had seen for check-ups; sent all his hygienist work to me when his hygienist left; gave me some of his nutty patients
- more introduction into oral surgery.

5 WHAT YOU HAVE LEARNT

What do you feel you have learnt most about in your first six months?

Answers:
- increasing speed; speed; to work faster
- running a practice
- coping with working under the NHS; the ins and outs of NHS regulations; what dentistry is like in the real NHS world
- increasing confidence; being able to cope with problems; feeling relaxed enough to question other practitioners on clinical problems without feeling inadequate
- most of the rules about covering yourself medico-legally
- treatment planning
- finance; profitable treatments.

Performance analysis

Reviewing the performance of the VDP by focusing on clinical outcomes and the processes that led to them is a useful technique, particularly in the early stages of training. It may take place by direct observation when opportunities arise, such as a request for assistance with a surgical extraction, by a record card review or during a problem-solving session during the tutorial. It can also take place through formal appraisal (*see* Appraisal).

Task analysis

This is carried out by first identifying individual tasks that the VDP would need to perform to bring out favourable clinical outcomes and to ascertain what knowledge and skills are required to perform those individual tasks. The aggregate of task components will affect overall performance. Task analysis is a useful tool in vocational training and is more fully discussed elsewhere in this book.

Competency studies

A competency study seeks to identify what knowledge and skills are required to demonstrate capability. Competence can be defined as 'the possession of the abilities required to manage a particular problem in a particular context' (Havelock *et al.*, 1995). Opportunities will arise during the training year to review how the VDP manages a variety of problems in a variety of contexts including the management of the individual patient in a variety of circumstances, and working within a team and within the wider context of the NHS regulations.

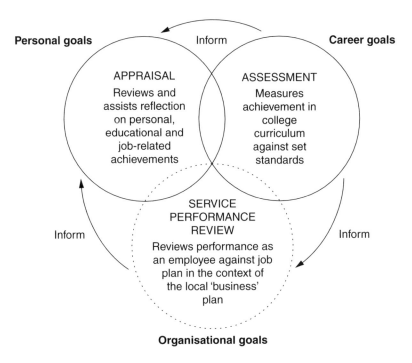

Figure 4.1 Relationships between appraisal, assessment and performance review (SCOPME, 1996).

Training needs survey

The purpose of the survey is to seek the collective and individual views of experienced trainers whose prior knowledge and experience of vocational training can help new trainers to gain a broad perspective on the likely training needs of recently qualified dentists.

Appraisal

The Standing Committee on Postgraduate Medical and Dental Education (SCOPME) defined appraisal as 'a confidential, educational review process for the benefit of the VDP' (SCOPME, 1996). It presented appraisal, assessment and performance review as a Venn diagram comprising three overlapping circles, each with its own characteristics and interlinked personal, career and organisational goals. It is a model that reflects the ethos of vocational training (Figure 4.1).

The key points to bear in mind about appraisal are:

- the appraisal interview should take place at a time convenient to the trainer and the VDP
- all the information should be at hand and performance review should take place against agreed criteria
- criticism should be constructive and through a process of self-realisation
- actions required to enhance future performance should be discussed and agreed.

There will be opportunities to carry out mini-appraisals throughout the early weeks in practice and the process will help to underpin future professional development plans.

It is interesting to compare the role of the trainer in these early weeks to that of a 'coach'. The most successful coaches have four core beliefs (Kinlaw, 1997):

1 people want to be successful; they want to do their best and bring credit upon themselves
2 people have a desire to learn and to perform
3 as people demonstrate competency, they want to become even more competent
4 when people are given the opportunity to demonstrate their competency, they will take that opportunity.

This should provide encouragement to trainers in those early weeks of practice with the VDP.

CHAPTER 5

Adult learning

The skills of teaching and training require an understanding of the key disciplines of adult learning. It is widely accepted that to be a good teacher requires far more than knowledge and experience and not all those who have expertise in any aspect of dentistry are able to teach effectively.

The essential skills include an ability to problem solve, present information in a structured and orderly fashion and communicate effectively. The extent of the learner's pre-existing knowledge, human motivation, and the impact of learning styles all play an important part in the teacher's approach to education.

Characteristics of adult learning

Vocational training is a form of self-directed adult learning. Self-directed learning 'describes a process in which individuals take the initiative, with or without the help of others, in diagnosing their learning needs, formulating learning goals, identifying human and material resources for learning, choosing and implementing appropriate learning strategies and evaluating learning outcomes' (Knowles, 1975). This definition is complex but comprehensive because it recognises the many facets of effective learning.

The simplest and earliest teaching/learning models relied heavily on teacher input. The teacher dictated what was learned, how it was learned, when it was learned and how the acquisition of knowledge was to be measured and tested in what became known as the pedagogical teaching model (pedagogy: from the Greek paid/agogus, meaning the art and science of teaching children). It was the dominant model in undergraduate teaching.

In contrast, the andragogical model focuses on helping adults learn. It is learner-sensitive and is the model of choice for the vocational training year.

Adult learning that involves VDPs differs in many respects. Brookfield (1986) has stated that adult learners are different because:

- they are not beginners, but are in a continuous process of growth and development
- they bring with them a set of experiences and values
- they arrive with an intention
- they have an expectation of the learning process
- they have competing interests – real-life events to contend with
- they already have their own pattern of learning.

There is no universally accepted approach to adult learning because of the diverse views amongst educationalists, but there are core themes and principles that trainers will find helpful. Trainers can assemble their training toolkit from these core principles.

Professional expertise in dentistry is one of those things that may be difficult to define in words but is easy to recognise in practice. It is made up of a number of elements (Figure 5.1).

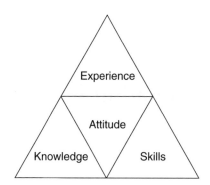

Figure 5.1 The elements of expertise.

Craft knowledge

The term 'craft knowledge' is particularly apt to dental vocational training. Craft knowledge refers to the processes of knowing what to do in a particular clinical situation, doing it and also examining how it was done. This combination of activity is what makes vocational training a unique learning environment because this type of training cannot be sought from a textbook. It is the sum of experience and actions moderated by good sense and judgement (Brown and McIntyre, 1993).

It is a reflection of the modesty of general practice trainers that they rarely appreciate the true value of their intellectual asset and it is this very asset that is called upon during the vocational training year.

In *The Reflective Practitioner*, the author notes:

even when a problem has been constructed it may escape the categories of applied science because it presents itself as unique or unstable ... a physician cannot apply standard techniques to a case that is not in the books (Schon, 1983).

The statement applies as much to dentistry as it does to the medical profession.

Craft knowledge is most evident during operative procedures in the form of fluency, the seamless execution of testing clinical procedures. This fluency, according to Schon, is facilitated by three factors:

1 selective information gathering – knowing what is relevant and what is not
2 the ability to minimise uncertainty
3 the ability to bring context into the decision-making process.

VDPs will require most assistance in these areas, and whilst solutions may appear 'obvious' to experienced trainers, a recent graduate raised on a diet of pedagogical teaching may experience difficulties.

Competence

Competence has been defined as 'the possession of the abilities required to manage a particular problem in a particular context' (Havelock *et al.*, 1995).

The main purpose of vocational training is to lead the VDP from a novice in general practice towards unsupervised practice. The work of Dreyfus and Dreyfus presents VT with a useful model that outlines a five-stage process to reflect the journey from novice to expert (Dreyfus and Dreyfus, 1984). Benner (whose eloquent summary is a pen picture of dental vocational training) has applied the approach very successfully to nursing:

> [The learner] *passes through five levels of proficiency: novice, advanced beginner, competent, proficient and expert. These different levels reflect changes in three general aspects of skilled performance. One is movement from reliance on abstract principles to the use of post-concrete experience as paradigms. The second is a change of the learner's perception of the demand situation, in which the situation is seen less and less as a compilation of equally relevant bits and more and more as a complete whole in which only certain parts are relevant. The third is a passage from detached observer to involved performer* (Benner, 1984).

Stage 4	Unconscious competence
Stage 3	Conscious competence
Stage 2	Conscious incompetence
Stage 1	Unconscious incompetence

Figure 5.2 Four stages: from novice to expert (Benner, 1984).

With this in mind, the typical pattern of progress of the inexperienced VDP can be summarised as shown in Figure 5.2. Many trainers believe that graduates straight from dental school join the VT scheme at stage 1, a stage at which they don't know what they don't know. The high-spirited confidence shown by some in the early days of practice is soon tempered by reality and stage 2 is quickly reached.

It is in stages 2 and 3 that the VDP is most vulnerable and needs most support and reassurance to help them move onto the next stage of their professional development.

Competence in general dental practice has additional elements to those considered in most definitions. These are summarised in Figure 5.3. The added dimensions in this cube are the elements of constraint, confluence and communication. Constraints arise from the limitations imposed on practitioners by regulatory narrative; confluence refers to the pooling of views and ideals from the peer group; and communication skills are essential interactive tools.

Bloom's taxonomy

In 1956 Benjamin Bloom and his team developed a classification of levels on intellectual behaviour that is important in education. This became a taxonomy that included three overlapping domains, all of which play a key part in vocational training. They are:

• cognitive – cognitive learning is demonstrated by knowledge recall

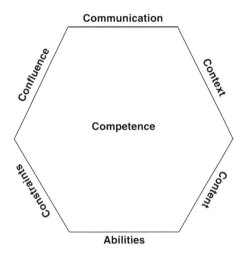

Figure 5.3 Facets of competence.

- affective – affective learning is demonstrated by behaviours that indicate attitudes and values
- psychomotor – demonstrated by co-ordination, dexterity, manipulation etc.

Within the cognitive domain, Bloom identified six levels ranging from the simple recall and recognition of facts to the highest order of evaluation. The six levels are shown in Figure 5.4.

With this structure in mind, trainers can base their training on the development of key abilities and attributes that can be summarised as follows:

- scientific knowledge
- diagnostic skills
- procedural skills
- problem solving
- decision making
- critical thinking
- interpersonal skills
- management skills
- professional attitudes and values.

Chapter 6 gives some examples of the teaching methods that can be used to develop these attributes.

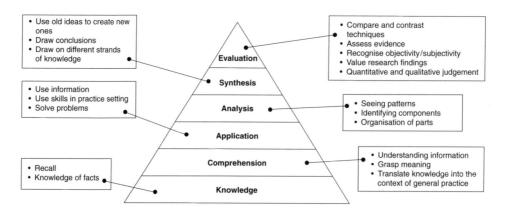

Figure 5.4 Bloom's taxonomy.

Learning styles

It has been long recognised that students have different preferences when it comes to the way they learn. Some prefer the formal setting of a lecture, some fare better in discussions groups and others respond better to personal study from textbooks. There are variations in study periods: some students prefer multiple short sessions, while others will study for hours and hours at a time. Some students perform better in the morning, some at night and some only when compelled to do so!

Four types of learning style have been identified (Honey and Mumford, 1986):

1 *the activist* – learning comes from new experiences and the activist is always asking 'what's new?'
2 *the reflector* – the reflector likes to think about things and reviews the task at hand
3 *the theorist* – theoretical models and an analytic approach dominate this style. The theorist will perform poorly unless he or she first has a conceptual framework to work with
4 *the pragmatist* – learning comes from the process of application. Linking theory and practice creates the best learning opportunities.

As an example, consider a new technique in endodontics – the use of nickel-titanium rotary files. The activist would be very excited by the new developments in technique and the motivation for learning would come from the 'newness' of the experience. The reflector would prefer to consider the new approach and give it some thought before embarking on the task. The theorist would want to know about instrument design and what advantages the technique offered over existing methods and would make analytic comparisons, whilst the pragmatist would have an understanding of the principles and learn by applying them at every opportunity.

All VDPs are different and trainers need to recognise that some styles work better in certain circumstances.

- *Activists* will learn best by 'being thrown in at the deep end' and from new situations and opportunities. They are always keen to 'have a go'. They sometimes over-stretch themselves and end up in situations they should have avoided. One example would be formulating over-ambitious treatment plans and then getting into clinical difficulties that required some hands-on help.
- *Reflectors* will need time to think and review before they perform and need to do this in their own time. New ideas and techniques should be introduced in a way that allows reflective VDPs time to absorb and think about them over a period of time before they will be ready to implement them. They will want to gather and share opinions and ideas and will not wish to be put under pressure. They are often methodical and thoughtful individuals. Reflectors sometimes frustrate their trainers because they are slow to act and make up their minds. They show hesitancy in treatment planning and may seek guidance from their trainers more often than their peers. Some patients may perceive this hesitancy and lack of assertiveness as inexperience or even incompetence.
- *Theorists* are best supported by facts and an intellectual approach to problem solving. They like to be stretched and to question and challenge ideas. They have a disciplined approach to treatment planning and are objective and analytical when dealing with clinical problems. The theorist can sometimes be too narrow-minded in their approach to clinical problem solving. They will not be comfortable with intuitive advice from their trainers but will quote from references, texts or undergraduate teachers.
- *Pragmatists* want lots of practical tips and hints. They like to watch procedures so they can pick up ideas that are not in the textbooks and will want to tap the trainer's experience. They are able to focus on practical aspects of dentistry. The pragmatist tends to reject anything that does not have a practical angle. They resist theory-based tutorial and do not perceive value in knowing anything unless they can apply their knowledge somewhere.

These styles of learning are not mutually exclusive. In reality individuals may lean towards a particular style, but there will probably also be evidence of elements typical of one or more of the other styles. The concept of learning styles does not promote singularity; on the contrary, co-existence can be a feature of the learning environment.

Another useful method is that proposed by Riding and Cheema (1991). The field dependence model is useful because it includes a number of key concepts, which are summarised in Box 5.1.

Box 5.1   Characteristics of field dependent/independent learners

Characteristics of field dependent learners

- Relate well to peer group.
- Use external frames of reference.
- Need external reinforcement.
- Need structured work.
- Good interpersonal skills.
- Need help with problem solving.

Characteristics of field independent learners

- Require little interaction with group.
- Use internal frame of reference.
- Intrinsic reinforcement.
- Structure own learning needs.
- Need help in developing social skills.
- Good at problem solving.

Patterns of learning

Learning curves are useful to demonstrate how the learning process takes place over time for different types of activity.

Figure 5.5a–d shows some examples of learning curves and their characteristics.

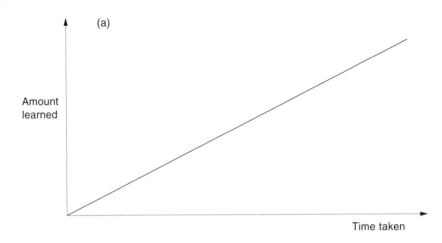

Figure 5.5a is a typical learning curve for a simple task. There is a linear relationship between the amount learned and the time taken. Such a curve would apply to explanations of practice procedures, simple clinical problems and how to overcome them etc.

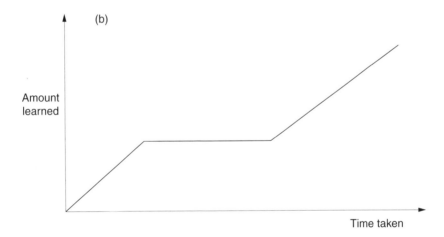

The pattern shown in **Figure 5.5b** is typical of difficult tasks, e.g. molar endodontics. It shows that the early teaching of the basic principles is fairly rapid because these have previously been taught at undergraduate level. At first, the curve rises steeply as new knowledge is introduced, but soon levels off because no further advancement can be made unless there is clinical experience to support it. The learning curve flattens with time once professional competence is reached. The boundaries of knowledge can always be extended by the very competent.

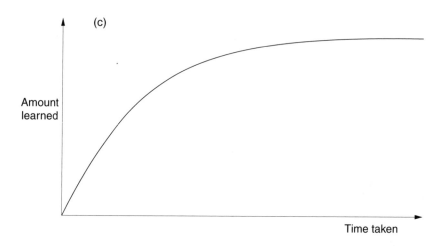

The trend shown in **Figure 5.5c** is typical of many VDPs in the early weeks of practice, and shows how the initial learning process takes place rapidly before reaching a plateau, and then rises in spurts over the first few weeks of training. The plateaux reflect periods of consolidation in the learning process.

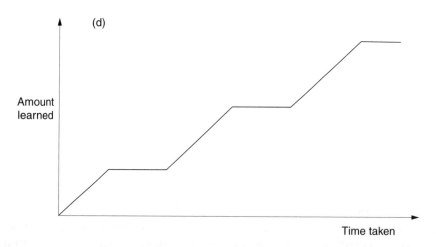

Figure 5.5d shows the form the curve takes during the course of the year with a series of small plateaux. Anecdotal evidence from many trainers suggests that VDPs experience the so-called 'mid-year blues' manifesting as a phase of inactivity, poor motivation and occasionally a *laissez-faire* approach to training. It is a phenomenon reported by many and probably represents an extended mid-year plateau. This may be due to a number of reasons that could include:

- a loss of trainer motivation
- a loss of VDP motivation
- an uninteresting or inappropriate subject
- distracting influences
- a dull teaching method
- no variety in teaching methods.

Attitudes in learning

Attitude has been defined as an individual's inclination to perceive and respond to events and situations in a characteristic manner. It features in the affective learning domain that was referred to in the discussion on Bloom's taxonomy.

Attitude influences learning behaviour. It is influenced by:

- peer group influences
- socio-economic environment
- the working environment
- professional past experiences
- personal past experiences.

Peer group influence
The VDP will be strongly influenced by the behaviour of his or her peers, i.e. other vocational VDPs. Trainers may wish to explore these influences with other trainers and the scheme organiser at the trainers' meetings.

The socio-economic environment
The environment in which the VDP has spent their formative years will affect their attitude towards certain things. This includes their domestic and educational environment.

The practice environment
The immediate working environment will influence the VDP's perceptions and colour their attitude.

Personal/professional past experiences
Traumatic personal and professional events can influence attitude formation. A VDP who has experienced early difficulties in oral surgery may have a negative attitude towards this subject. In practice, this may become evident if the VDP insists on referring all such procedures.

Attitude change

Trainers must accept that there will be differences between their own attitudes towards certain things and those of their VDPs. If these differences are a threat to the VDP's professional development, it becomes part of the trainer's responsibility to try and change the attitude.

This change in attitude could be brought about by peer group pressure or by input from an influential colleague. Peer group pressure might originate from other VDPs on the VT scheme. Trainers can question their VDPs about how fellow VDPs feel about a particular situation or set of circumstances or how they react in a given situation. By exploring peer attitudes, individual VDPs are often inspired to change their own.

The influence of a highly regarded or more experienced colleague, who could be another dentist within the practice, can also exert a positive influence on someone's poor attitude towards some aspect of practice.

If trainers have particular concerns about poor attitude that prove difficult to resolve, the VT adviser should be informed and it may be that particular issues can be addressed through general discussions during the study days. Any change in attitude resulting from this approach would indirectly be an example of peer group pressure.

Useful concepts

The processes through which learning takes place are summarised in Table 5.1. The 'areas of training' identified in this table are all facets of vocational training in general dental practice.

Table 5.1   Some examples of broad-based concepts and how they relate to VT in general practice

Process	What it means and how it works	Areas of training
Osmosis	Peer group influence, particularly relevant in discussions on the VT study days and with other colleagues	Group dynamics
Symbiosis	The importance of developing and encouraging mutually beneficial relationships	Team building in the practice environment
Homeostasis	Individuals wanting to revert to type during times of change; they will want to maintain the status quo at all costs and may hinder development	Change management; responding to changes in system; coping with trends
Mind–body linkages	The importance of keeping physically fit; the healthy mind/healthy body concept; sometimes called 'psycho-physical dualism' (for those who like jargon!)	Stress management; anxiety control
Capacity building	The process of helping someone who, as a result of that help, develops the capacity to help themselves; reflects ethos of VT	Helping to create the self-managed learner

CHAPTER 6

Teaching methods

A variety of teaching methods are used in vocational training and many of them relate to aspects of adult learning that were covered in the previous chapter.

The range of approaches to effective learning is summarised below. (Kolb *et al.*, 1974). They describe these as:

- **experiential** – learning by doing
- **participative** – involving the learner as much as possible
- **instructional** – learning in stages
- **didactic** – syllabus-based learning.

Within this framework, experiential learning is the cornerstone of vocational training. The process of experiential learning is best illustrated in the experiential learning cycle (Figure 6.1).

The objectives of experiential learning are summarised in Table 6.1.

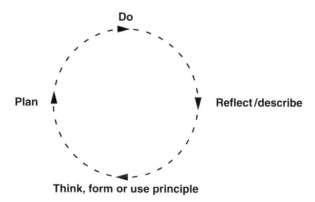

Figure 6.1 The experiential learning cycle.

Table 6.1 Objectives of experiential learning

Objective	Comments
Affective objectives	Affective processes bring about changes in feelings, attitudes and values and, as a result, can influence behaviour and how situations and circumstances are perceived.
Empathic objectives	Empathy is concerned with shared feelings and being able to see things from someone else's perspective. In dental practice this often means seeing things from a patient's perspective or taking into account a fellow team member's viewpoint. Having empathic objectives is part of learning to work as part of a team.
Interactive objectives	This involves the acquisition of new skills such as interviewing, handling difficult situations, including complaints, and coping with challenging clinical situations.
Unlearning objectives	Often misunderstood, this relates to the unlearning of prejudices, stereotype ideals and other psychological impediments in favour of an unbiased perspective.
Higher level cognitive skills	High level skills including sensory motor skills can be acquired and practised until they can be delivered with fluency.

Teaching styles

The Royal College of General Practitioners, in one of the first published works on teaching in general practice, proposed a variety of teaching styles that were tutor-focused (Royal College of General Practitioners, 1972):

- **authoritarian** – the teacher states the fact but discourages questions. This is an appropriate style for delivering a list of facts
- **socratic** – this is a question and answer style. The tutor does the asking and the learner does the responding and the session evolves as the learners demonstrate lack of knowledge in particular areas
- **heuristic** – this is learning by adopting a doing/discovery approach where the learner takes total responsibility. It has some similarities with problem-based learning, *see* Chapter 7.

- **counselling** – this is a softer, less defined approach that relies on ascertaining the reasons for the learner's ignorance.

The development of in-practice training should be a seamless continuum of processes that comprise one or more of the following:

- problem-based learning
- direct observation
- task analysis
- case studies
- video and CD-ROM
- practice meetings
- in-practice referrals
- tutorials
- access to e-learning opportunities.

Problem-based learning

Problem-based learning opportunities arise frequently in the early months of the training year. The triggers are usually one or more of the following:

- VDP requests hands-on help in a particular clinical situation
- patient returns after treatment with complications
- patient complains about some aspect of the treatment
- unsuccessful treatment outcomes.

Typical examples would be a request for assistance with an oral surgery procedure, the development of an acute problem following treatment, adverse comments by a patient to a member of staff or a failed post crown. Each of these is an example of each of the categories listed above and presents trainers and VDPs with valuable teaching opportunities.

Problem-based learning is covered more fully in Chapter 7.

Direct observation

Widely used in undergraduate teaching, direct observation is a good way to teach and demonstrate practical skills and the use of equipment and instruments.

The demonstration is based on the 'you do as I do' principle. The easiest way for trainees to observe is to act as dental assistant to the trainer during clinical procedures.

For the best results using this method, the following key points should be borne in mind:

• allow sufficient time for procedure and commentary
• select a willing and co-operative patient
• discuss and plan the proposed treatment before starting
• explain the rationale for each stage.

This approach is illustrated in the following example.

Example: The direct observation of a surgical extraction of a buried root.

Key areas for discussion would include:

• flap design
• raising the flap – technique and common errors
• bone removal – technique, choice of instruments and how to use them
• elevation of root – choice of elevator, design and method of application
• wound closure
• postoperative procedures.

Task analysis

This involves a step-by-step analysis of any clinical procedure. The analysis should include a summary of:

• what you, as the trainer, normally do
• what your trainee was taught to do
• an overview of the alternatives
• a review of the literature.

This process is ideal for discussing more complex procedures.

A sectional analysis technique is frequently used. This involves the subdivision of a procedure into smaller units, followed by an analysis of each in turn, as in the example shown in Box 6.1 involving molar endodontics. This procedure, which is identified frequently as an area for concern amongst VDPs, lends itself to discussion in segments because attention can be focused on any particular aspect of the task. Practical demonstrations accelerate the learning process and thus improve the quality of training. In this example, the procedures may be first demonstrated on an extracted tooth prior to a chairside demonstration.

Box 6.1 Molar endodontics in stages

Gaining access	Access cavity design in relation to internal and external tooth morphology. Choice of burs. Gauging depth. Avoiding complications such as perforations. Use of instruments, e.g. DG16 explorers.
Preparation, shaping and cleansing	Initial access. Step back vs. step down techniques. Coronal flaring. Use/choice of irrigants. Irrigation techniques. Ultrasonics. Choice of instruments including use of NiTi rotary files. Avoiding complications. Working length determination. Apex locators.
Obturation	Conventional techniques. Choice of instruments. Thermoplastic options. Use and choice of root canal sealers. Postoperative assessment.

Case studies

Case studies are a practical and useful training tool. A variety of cases should be selected to illustrate the diversity of clinical conditions and the prescribed treatment.

Case analysis by treatment type
The selection of a specific case to illustrate one type of treatment is a simple example and a useful prompt for a discussion later. Either the trainer or the trainee, both of whom should be prepared to give their views, may select the case. Conflicting clinical opinions are a part of professional practice and can form the basis of reasoned and challenging discussions, but care should be taken that they do not lead to interpersonal conflict.

Case analysis by random selection
Random selection and perusal of patient record cards can stimulate discussions on a variety of topics. There is no time for advance preparation, but in-depth discussions can be scheduled for a later date if the analysis has revealed a subject of particular interest. Remember that even the simplest of treatment plans can generate plentiful discussion and expose variations in treatment philosophies.

Problem case analysis

Trainers are encouraged to present their own problem cases, both past and present, and not to rely solely on the trainee's input. It is important that trainees are aware that all clinicians, however experienced, have to contend with difficulties and failures.

Ideally, the discussion of a problem case should take place fairly soon after the problem has been identified.

Video and CD-ROM

Videotapes and CD-ROM are now widely available and many practices will have copies in the practice library for trainees to access. Video is a useful teaching tool and provides an added stimulus to the training programme.

Again, preparation is important, and the content should be used to generate critical discussion. Video may be used in association with other training techniques, for example to enhance case discussions, and/or to become part of a task analysis exercise.

Practice meetings

Practice meetings provide valuable training and learning opportunities. The VDP is probably better placed to contribute in a meaningful way in the second half of the training year rather than at the beginning. Invite the VDP to participate in the discussions and involve them in the final decision-making process.

In-practice referrals

If a practice colleague has a special interest in any particular aspects of dentistry, invite them to participate in the training programme. VDPs can only benefit from this additional exposure to professional expertise. Some trainers will encourage their VDP to visit and spend sessions with neighbouring practitioners, to whom they may refer, to extend the range and quality of clinical experience.

Tutorials

A tutorial is a period of individual tuition between the trainer and the VDP. It makes a significant contribution to the VDP's professional development. The aims of the tutorial session are:

- to discuss specific case histories and treatment planning issues
- to solve problems that may have arisen
- to impart knowledge about the rationale for treatment techniques
- to learn about practice management and related subjects
- to develop existing skills and acquire new ones
- to support the VDP in his or her personal and professional development.

Trainers and VDPs are expected to devote at least one hour each week to tutorial tuition and to keep a record of their discussions in the professional development portfolio. The tutorial should take place during the working day and in protected time, free from interruptions and outside distraction.

This contractual requirement remains in force for the entire duration of the vocational training period.

Many of these are two-way interactions such as discussions, problem solving and counselling. Others, such as teaching, are normally trainer-led processes which, in order to be effective, should address the needs and wants of the VDP.

Conducting a tutorial

The tutorial is the backbone of in-practice teaching and training. To deliver effective and interesting tutorials, trainers should focus not only on the content, but also on the process of delivery. *See* Appendix 3 for a list of some of the many topics suitable for discussion during tutorials.

For maximum impact, effective tutorials will require:

- preparation
- planning
- priorities
- participation.

Preparation

Decide in advance which subject(s) will be covered during the tutorial session. Both trainers and VDPs should prepare the subject(s) beforehand to ensure the discussions are as productive as possible.

Try to use audio-visual aids, such as models, radiographs, videos, literature, slides etc., which can stimulate discussions and add another dimension to the tutorial. The audio-visual materials must be available at the start of the tutorial so that valuable time is not lost during the session looking for the key items.

The physical layout of the room in which the tutorials are held is an important consideration. Chairs should have open space between them, or be placed next to each other one side of a desk. This is important to encourage discursive tutorials.

Planning

Whenever possible, trainers should use practice resources. The wealth of knowledge and expertise within the practice can provide much of the material for planning and conducting effective tutorials.

If clinical techniques are discussed, these discussions should centre on cases that have been treated or are currently under treatment in the practice. This is one of the main roles of the trainer – to provide on-site, hands-on practical teaching and training. This approach is considered to be far more beneficial than the method of simply going through a series of revised lecture notes that the trainer may have acquired. The notes may form the basis of discussion, or they may be used as support material, but they should not be used to deliver a lecture to what is, in effect, an audience of one.

Plan and structure the tutorial around the time available, allowing sufficient time for discussion and demonstration. Lack of material to fill the time available is as much a sign of poor planning as overloading the session with too much information.

Always plan to keep something in reserve in case there is time left at the end. Discussions centred on new materials or instruments are very useful 'fillers' to slot in if time allows.

Tutorial design is also a part of the planning process. The tripartite approach, a simple but effective way of designing a tutorial, can be applied to most situations.

With a tripartite approach, the tutorial is divided into three time blocks, each of, say, 20 minutes duration, although the exact division of time will depend on what is planned for the session.

Specific topics can then be explored in each time block, or, in the case of more complex topics, one block might be allocated for analysis, another for a hands-on demonstration, and the last for the questions and answers.

Example: Fabrication of composite inlays.

Part 1: Discussion of the technique including an overview of clinical indications and limitations of the technique. Case selection, with examples of patients from the practice.

Part 2: Table demonstration of preparation technique, handling of materials and/or video presentation of the technique. Discussion of clinical and laboratory procedures involved.
Part 3: Assessing the procedure. Common pitfalls to avoid. Questions and answers and debrief.

In this way a tutorial can be structured to include one or more topics that would come under the following headings:

• clinical
• professional/ethical
• administration
• personal/social
• managerial.

With thoughtful planning, an opportunity could be made available for the trainee to assist the trainer in just such a clinical procedure on a patient, thus providing an excellent opportunity to reinforce many of the key points covered in the tutorial.

Advance planning involves trainee participation. If a tutorial is planned on a particular subject, the trainee should be given a task to prepare for the tutorial in advance. This could be anything from reading around the subject, or gathering information on an innovative product.

Priorities
The tutorial should be a learner-centred activity. Decide what the trainee wants to discuss and what is most important to him or her on that day. Be prepared to give spontaneous tutorials. It may be that a particular clinical or administrative problem demands immediate attention and this would then take priority over the planned tutorial topic.

Participation
The participative style is the style of choice for the majority of tutorials. It encourages trainee involvement from the outset and places the correct emphasis on joint preparation. It is also a style that encourages the development of professional rapport between trainer and trainee.

Table 6.2 Favoured qualities in trainer teaching styles

Friendly	*Organised*	*Stimulating*
• warm	• responsible	• imaginative
• understanding	• business-like	• ambitious
• approachable	• systematic	• motivated

Research into tutorial styles has shown that learners favour tutors who have certain characteristics. These are summarised in Table 6.2.

This ten-point checklist was put forward at one of the many centrally-held workshops organised and run by CVT to assist new trainers. It summarises much of what has been discussed in this chapter:

1 look back, here and now, look forward (reflect and plan)
2 what's on top? (prioritise)
3 let VDP prompt first
4 get them talking and working
5 tasks and reading are okay
6 use artefacts, checklists, visual material
7 use the learning cycle – experience, reflection, thinking, planning
8 link experience to topic: past and 'what if'
9 negotiate: content and process
10 next week: next tutorial . . .

Common errors
New trainers often express reservations about their ability to conduct tutorials. The proper emphasis on processes, planning and participation will all facilitate the trainer's task. The common errors to avoid when giving a tutorial are:

- *The monologue*: The trainer simply delivers a lecture. There is no exchange of information or feedback from the trainee.
- *Interrogation*: The tutorial becomes a question-and-answer session with the trainer asking a series of rapid-fire questions often in a random and illogical sequence.
- *Diversion*: Distractions that sway one or other of the two parties' concentration from the mainstream subject render the entire exercise futile.
- *Hurrying*: This arises when insufficient time is allowed to discuss a subject in the depth it deserves. The trainer is tempted to skip through information quickly and the trainee has insufficient time to absorb it.

If the trainer avoids falling into any of these traps, both parties can reap the benefits of a constructive and well-designed tutorial.

e-learning

The American Society for Training and Development has defined e-learning as 'anything delivered, enabled or mediated by electronic technology for the explicit purpose of learning'. It is more than computer-based learning. Examples of e-learning include:

- on-line discussion groups
- web-based chat rooms
- video-conferencing by computer
- receiving e-mail from a tutor, mentor or colleague.

The society has been closely involved in the development of many innovative e-learning initiatives and uses the acronym FIRST to set out its e-learning criteria, which are:

- *Fast* – programme design and development within two months or less.
- *Inexpensive* – how much will it cost and can the material be used in other ways?
- *Relative* – who is the learner?
- *Simple* – do we have the skills and tools to do the job?
- *Trackable* – did the learner receive training and how can we measure what was learned?

This is a very useful list of criteria to govern the design of e-learning initiatives. There are currently several such initiatives in the pipeline in the UK. At the time of writing, it is very likely that one or two dominant organisations or individuals will emerge as market leaders in this new and exciting field but there is still much development work to be done.

The advantages of e-learning are that it allows practices to take full advantage of existing computers and networks to access information from a number of sites. It may be looked upon as a development of correspondence and distance learning courses. In general terms, the advantages of e-learning are:

- *Convenience* – access on demand means that the learner is not limited by time and place constraints and learning takes place at a time convenient to the learner.
- *Efficient mode of information transmission* – information is readily available to view on-line, to download or save in a chosen file format. The process is quick, easy and user friendly.
- *Interactive opportunities* – the integration of text, images, audio and video can make e-learning vivid and stimulate the learner. Interaction can also be enhanced through the use of various e-tools. These include e-mail, which is an efficient way of exchanging messages, bulletin boards, which provide a forum for discussion and can encourage critical reflection, chat rooms, which allow real time discussion of current

issues and various home pages, which list resources and offer links to other opportunities.

- *Modifications to course material are easier* – material can be easily changed and updated to ensure that it reflects current trends.
- *Potential cost savings* – there are direct and indirect financial benefits. There is no need to produce and mail documents, therby reducing stationery and postage costs. Indirect cost savings include time saved on travelling and searching for information.
- *Knowledge transference* – facts, figures and other cognitive elements can be delivered very effectively.

In addition, there are many new initiatives planned for the dental professional that will emerge in the near future and it is likely that trainers will have access to an increasing number of e-resources in the future.

However, there are some disadvantages, which include:

- *Technology fear* – fear of the new technology and a reluctance to accept a changing climate can impede learning. This is more likely to apply to trainers than to VDPs, the majority of whom have access to and have regularly used technology during their undergraduate studies.
- *Networking costs* – the infrastructure can be expensive to install and frequent upgrades may be required to keep pace with software and other technological advances. Downloads can be time consuming unless there is access to special lines that allow for rapid access.
- *Interaction* – Just as e-learning offers interactive opportunities, it denies the learner direct human contact. This can impede the learning process.
- *Development costs* – costs vary but estimates between £10 000–£15 000 per hour of content are not uncommon.

There is no doubt that e-learning will have some impact on the future of education. John Chambers, CEO of Cisco Systems, famously commented during a 1999 conference, that 'there will be two great equalisers in life going forward – the Internet and education, and they must go hand in hand'.

The extent of the likely impact of e-learning on dental vocational training is difficult to predict. Undoubtedly, there will be initial euphoria of information access, and video-streaming opportunities will doubtless excite technophiles, but there is more to training than information access. Inspiration, role modelling, enthusiasm and motivation all play an important part in the education process, and electronic transmission does not necessarily create an environment within which this can flourish. It can be argued that the medium lessens the impact of the message when the target audience is deprived of the human interactions, which facilitate and underpin the learning process.

The e-revolution is happening and future development is inevitable. It is unlikely to replace the face-to-face interactions that create synergy within the learning environment totally, but it will undoubtedly become an important part in the future of vocational training. For example, it is possible to run e-learning sessions with a speaker and a virtual classroom tool, which allows live sessions to be run across the internet or intranet.

It is worth noting that the quality of on-line learning is only as good as the copywriters and designers who created it. In this sense it is no different from the face-to-face methods.

Conclusions

It has been said that 20% of what we read we recall, 30% of what we hear we recall, 40% of what we see we recall, 50% of what we say we recall and 90% of what we see, hear, say and do, we recall. This summarises the preferred teaching methods used in the practice during the vocational training year.

Teaching methods are enhanced by:

- setting goals and targets
- dividing subject matter into small learning units
- teaching practical skills in sequence
- repeating as often as needed
- checking understanding frequently before advancing
- increasing learner motivation.

Teaching methods are less effective when:

- insufficient opportunities are available to practise new skills
- there is a lack of opportunity to apply new knowledge
- there is a poor understanding of basic concepts
- there are conflicting views on techniques
- key points are not repeated.

Comparisons between conventional teaching methods and on-line initiatives show that the former are not necessarily better or worse than the latter; they are just different. On e-learning, Eaton (2001) gives a pragmatic and relevant perspective:

> *An on-line programme is very unlikely to meet the needs of those completely new to any profession. This is because novices will not have*

any basis in practical experience or personal insight needed to convert the materials on the screen into new skills. However, once some work experience has been gathered, the platform can appear for reflection and re-conceptualisation that is essential to learning.

One perspective of the future is shown in Figure 6.2.

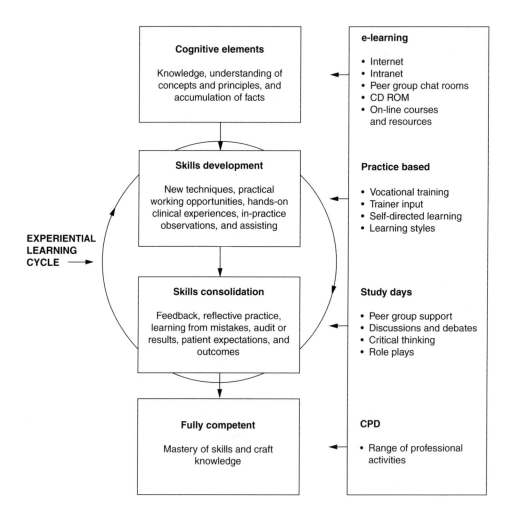

Figure 6.2   Proposal for a training management system.

CHAPTER 7

Problem-based learning

Although problem-based learning (PBL) has received much publicity in recent years, the concept is far from new; it has been successfully used in some American medical schools for over 25 years. It began at McMaster University Medical School and has since been implemented in many undergraduate and postgraduate education programmes throughout the world.

In 1990, a new undergraduate dental curriculum was introduced in Malmo that was based almost entirely on PBL. It promoted a holistic care approach to the treatment of patients in which basic sciences and clinical dentistry were integrated to create a new approach to dental training.

The PBL pathway is best suited to individuals who:

- are self-directed
- are comfortable with flexibility and ambiguity in their learning role
- learn best through discussion and reading
- want a strong clinical context for their learning.

What is PBL?

PBL is an educational strategy that promotes active learning and has its roots in cognitive psychology. A detailed discussion falls outside the scope of this book, but it may be helpful to outline briefly the three key factors in this particular learning process. They are:

- the activation of prior knowledge
- encoding specificity
- the elaboration of knowledge.

A 'problem' can best be thought of as 'a goal where the correct path to its solution is not known' (*see* www.pbli.org).

Activation of prior knowledge

It is the extent of prior knowledge that affects an individual's ability to acquire new knowledge. The trainer's task is to activate this prior knowledge in the context of the general practice environment.

Anecdotal evidence suggests that many trainers feel that VDPs are ill prepared for general practice, despite protestations to the contrary by their undergraduate teachers! There may be many reasons for these different perceptions, but one significant factor is the environment in which the knowledge is activated and put to the test. The requirements of dental school are very different from the demands of general practice and this is essentially what creates the conflicting perceptions of competence.

Encoding specificity

This concerns the processes of information storage and retrieval. It has been shown that the context in which something is learned (context specificity) has a strong impact on how that information is then later retrieved (processing specificity).

It is known that the closer the learning experience to the situation in which the information will be used, the better the performance of that individual. The corollary to this is that the creation of similar learning and application environments favours encoding specificity. Therein lies the value of vocational training because the education is taking place in the very environment where it will be used.

The use of simulators, in training pilots for example, is an excellent example of what is sometimes referred to as 'learning in a functional concept'.

Elaboration of knowledge

The process of understanding is enhanced when the learner is able to add to existing knowledge through peer group discussions. This is called the process of elaboration, and it closely reflects what takes place at the practice as well as on the study course during the VT year.

Key features

The principles of PBL should be known to VDPs in order to prepare them for effective life-long learning in a profession where the emergence of new techniques and the re-evaluation of existing ones underpins the practice of evidence-based dentistry. (There is an old educational truism that sums this up. It states that half of what students are taught is out of date by the time they enter the real world and no-one can accurately predict which half that will be.)

In PBL, it is the VDP who assumes the greater responsibility for learning. This approach increases motivation and heightens feelings of achievement. PBL and VT fit well together because they share some common features. These include:

• learner centredness
• learning occurs in the practice environment
• the trainer is the facilitator
• the focus of learning is an identified problem
• it prepares participants to be life-long learners.

The PBL approach is a particularly effective means of delivering in-practice training because a lot of clinical reasoning is essentially a problem-solving process. PBL is now a widely used tool in many undergraduate teaching programmes because it has a number of advantages over conventional, more didactic teaching methods.

In one recent study, which explored the use of PBL in vocational training (Mowat and Stewart, 1999), trainers considered it to be 'worthwhile, enjoyable, good, dynamic and interesting' and noted that:

• it allowed exploration of issues that could not readily be covered by a more traditional format
• it provided opportunities for applying theoretical knowledge to real-life situations
• it signalled a welcome move away from the 'spoon-fed' approach to a more independent mode of learning and thinking
• it helped VDPs to identify their own learning goals.

The PBL approach is best summarised in the 5-step sequence shown in Figure 7.1

In this sequence, the trainer's role is to facilitate and to provide input at key stages. The trainer may design and provide simulated problems that will challenge the VDP and encourage him or her to develop problem-solving skills. It is important that this sequence takes place within the context of reflective learning.

The outcome of these discussions will help to put the experience in the context of everyday practice with all the ethical dilemmas that poses. This creates what has been described as a 'multi-pathway' model, which relies

1   Learner confronts a problem

2   Learner organises pre-existing knowledge and attempts to identify the nature of the problem

3   Learner/trainer discuss the problem

4   Learner identifies the resources required to solve the problem

5   Information is gathered with input from the trainer in an attempt to solve the problem

Figure 7.1   The five-step sequence for PBL.

heavily on effective and frequent communication between the VDP and the trainer and which is facilitated by maintaining an 'open door' policy at the practice. A good example of the 'multi-pathway' model is the scenario of discussing the potential problems associated with the complication of a separated endodontic instrument. Discussions would need to consider reasons for separation, avoidance of recurrence, correct/incorrect use of instruments, design of instruments, retrieval options, referral protocols, possible clinical sequelae, medico-legal implications, communication skills and financial implications.

In this way, PBL has been defined as both a curriculum and a process (*see* www.pbli.org).

Key components

The key components of PBL are as follows.

VDPs must have responsibility for their own learning

This has been emphasised in other chapters and is also a key element of PBL. Not all VDPs will be familiar with a PBL approach to education and many will have been taught with a very traditional didactic approach. At a recent regional induction day, 51 VDPs were asked to complete a questionnaire to gain a better understanding of their baseline expectation. One of the sections of the questionnaire posed the question 'Who do you think is responsible for your professional development this year?'. They were given a range of possible answers, all of which cited the trainer, the VDP and the scheme adviser, but which attached different weightings to each. Almost 80% of respondents placed 70% of the responsibility for learning with the trainer or scheme adviser and only 30% with themselves.

VDPs must be taught how to decide what they need to know and should be guided by their trainers into seeking appropriate resources, including books, journals, on-line resources and the experience of their peers. This emphasises that PBL is essentially a VDP-centred activity and that the trainer's role is largely facilitatory.

Problem simulations should be deliberately ill-structured

This aspect of PBL may appear to contradict one of the edicts of vocational training, which is to plan and be well prepared for tutorials. In reality, there is no conflict here because problem simulations should be planned, but they should be planned to be in an unstructured format. This encourages lateral thinking and does not restrict the scope of the inquiry into the simulation.

Learning should be integrated with a broad spectrum of subjects

This allows for all aspects of a problem to be fully discussed and helps the VDP to put clinical situations into the wider context of general practice and the social environment. A typical clinical problem, for example, could lead to broader discussions that include:

- record keeping
- patient management and communication skills
- psychology of dental care
- medico-legal consequences
- business implications.

Collaboration is helpful

Many VT study days on the course begin with a problem-solving session, which provides VDPs with a valuable opportunity to discuss situations with their peers. This type of collaborative work is a valuable part of the day and an integral component of PBL because it gives them confidence, authority and responsibility for their own development. It also provides opportunities to rehearse the skills that they will routinely use as members of a practice team.

Application and resolution

There should be evidence of understanding and application of problem-solving techniques in everyday practice. The VDP should then be better able to deal with any similar situations that may arise.

Closing analysis

There should be an opportunity for VDPs to analyse the outcomes of their deliberations. They should be able to reflect on what they have learned and how this knowledge will help them to cope with any similar situations that arise. The closing analysis is a summary of their thoughts and it helps to identify and categorise, in some order of preference or priority, all the discussions that have taken place. It helps to create a shift from what has been described as procedural knowledge to declarative knowledge, which can be applied at a later date.

Self-assessment

The VDP should be able to recognise his or her professional development as a result of this training methodology. The professional development portfolio is one vehicle for achieving this. It is a means of providing feedback. Trainers should also provide verbal feedback to VDPs because evidence is emerging that suggests the outcomes of a PBL approach are having a direct impact on the clinical and managerial performance of the VDP.

The activities and simulations must relate to the real world

Simulations must also mirror real-life situations to ensure that the activities and processes undertaken to solve a problem have lasting value and can be applied to real-life situations at a later date. Situations that are perceived as unlikely or far-fetched will not be taken seriously and the benefits of the process will be limited.

PBL should be part of everyday in-practice teaching

The advocates of PBL emphasise that it should be a way of life in the practice teaching environment and not simply a bolt-on extra to traditional didactic methods. Many aspects of traditional memory-based teaching conflict with the principles of PBL and it is important to establish the new focus at an early stage of the training year, particularly where the graduates have not been exposed to a PBL approach at undergraduate level.

Problem-solving styles

It has been shown that individuals demonstrate three problem-solving styles (Cox and Ewan, 1988).

1 Pattern recognition
Clinical training and experiences are stored as a bank of clinical patterns. VDPs will recognise these patterns in the first few minutes of a consultation; if this doesn't happen in the early stages, then it probably won't happen at all. This 'recognition' process is directly proportional to knowledge and experience, and the trainer can 'imprint' these patterns on the VDP to facilitate recognition.

2 Diagnosis-directed search
If there is no pattern, then the VDP enters 'search mode'. This is an analytical approach and relies on the 'accumulation' of data to deduce the solution. Trainers can facilitate the process by addressing any knowledge deficit and encouraging critical thinking.

3 Systematic enquiry
This is the process of 'history-taking', which VDPs have been taught at undergraduate level. Trainers can facilitate this process by letting the VDP observe them in consultation with patients presenting with complex symptoms.

Conclusions

A review of the literature is generally supportive of PBL as an educational strategy in health-oriented professions. The idea of engaging the learner has now been tried and tested in many medical and dental institutions with great success and it continues to evolve.

It has been shown that learners exposed to the methods of PBL have become proficient in problem solving, self-directed learning and team participation. They have been shown to have acquired the knowledge, skills and attitudes at least as well as those trained in the conventional way, but have become better practitioners of their profession.

The outcomes of PBL have been identified as:

- problem-solving skills
- self-directed learning skills
- critical thinking
- self-motivation
- leadership skills
- communication skills
- proactive thinking
- congruence with workplace skills.

(*see* www.samford.edu/pbl)

All of these are important elements of the VT year.

CHAPTER 8

Small group teaching

Trainers are encouraged to contribute to the small group teaching sessions on the study days. The combination of theoretical knowledge, understanding and general practice experience makes trainers a natural choice for inclusion in the course programme. However, a lack of teaching experience dissuades many from contributing to the study days. Trainers who are reluctant to participate cite common concerns such as:

> *I've never done anything like this before. What if they don't like me?*
> *I think they probably know more than I do.*
> *What if I dry up in the middle of the presentation?*
> *I don't think I have enough material to run an entire session.*
> *I don't have any audio-visual material.*

Many of these comments reflect a fear of failure and lack of confidence, but all these concerns can be overcome with a little help and guidance from colleagues and the scheme adviser. Small group teaching is a skill, and like all skills it has to be rehearsed to be effective. Some regions organise short courses on teaching and presentation skills, but there is no substitute for direct hands-on involvement. *See* Chapter 9 for a discussion about presentation skills.

The majority of teaching in vocational training takes place at small group level. There are a number of advantages to this, which include the following:

- it encourages involvement of all group members
- it encourages the pooling of experience and information
- there is ample scope for developing a dynamic relationship and many presenters 'get to know' their groups within a relatively short time
- there are opportunities for learning from one's peers as individuals feel more confident to express their views
- group members can offer mutual support.

These are important features of group work and are advantageous because they help to optimise learning. Without them, a postgraduate training programme would be akin to distance learning.

Small groups

The effectiveness of small group teaching is related to group size, which can vary from year to year. Its main aim is to develop and to explore professional competencies.

To facilitate this process, consider the following:

- ground rules
- seating positions
- group size.

Ground rules

Explain the ground rules at the beginning of the session.

- Advise the group if you are happy for members to interrupt you at any stage, or whether you prefer to leave questions until the end.
- Establish the protocol for interruptions and group work.
- Inform the group of your expectations, and elicit from them what they expect of you, and what they hope to gain from your presentation.
- Establish 'margins of safety'. Individual group members should feel sufficiently at ease to express their views without embarrassment or criticism from either the speaker or the remainder of the group.
- Give an indication of tasks and timings.
- Remember the techniques of risk reduction and reward.

Risk reduction is achieved by setting tasks that lie within the capability of the group, by stating clear aims and objectives and by avoiding criticism of incorrect statements or illogical arguments. Always maintain a courteous and caring approach, no matter how absurd the input from individual members.

Efforts should be rewarded initially by acknowledgement, and then by an invitation to continue the theme of the response. This introduces the all-important 'feel good' factor, which remains a key issue in the perceived educational value of the session.

Seating positions

The physical relationship between the teacher and the group has a remarkable influence on the type of interactions that take place during the presentation.

Figure 8.1a–d shows three common configurations. The arrows indicate the likely communication processes amongst members. Some configurations encourage more participation than others. The least participative is the configuration shown in Figure 8.1a, which is tutor dominated and tends to exclude group members seated at the rear, particularly those in the rear corners.

The seating arrangement shown in Figure 8.1b will encourage more involvement between members seated next to each other and between them and the tutor. This particular configuration favours tasks that are set for pairs because trainees are able to face each other with minimum disruption to the overall seating plan.

In the arrangement shown in Figure 8.1c the main group has been split into three sub-groups. This facilitates inter- and intra-group participation.

The nature and style of presentation will determine the optimum seating position and presenters should consider the configurations as part of their presentation planning process. The configuration can be changed at any time thereafter to suit the activity, delivery and content of the presentation. The physical shifting of position is in itself a non-verbal cue as to the intended interactions.

The configuration shown in Figure 8.1d is often known as 'the fish bowl'. It is a group-on-group configuration in which the inner group (A) is given a task to discuss and the outer group (B) act as observers. At the end of the task time, the outer group would be expected to report on their observations and are permitted to add their own observations on the assignment.

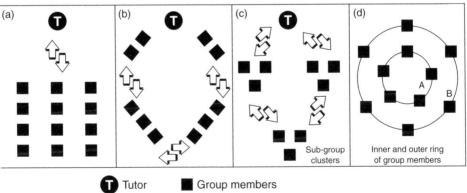

Figure 8.1a–d Examples of seating configurations.

'The fish bowl' is ideal for a number of worthwhile exercises. Examples include:

- *problem solving* – one group listening to another encourages a high level of participation
- *to stimulate divergent views* – inner and outer group members can be selected for their known and different perspectives to encourage divergent views. A trainer who presents on the course would not necessarily be aware of these views, and some advance preparation with the VT adviser can be useful
- *to observe group behaviour* – it helps to identify the dynamic pathways within the group.

Group size

The general view is that the optimum group size consists of approximately 12 individuals. Sub-division of the main group into smaller units is one way of maximising participation from members of the group for any particular task. Small group interactions are perceived as less threatening and allow individuals to express themselves within the privacy of limited numbers.

Group dynamics

Much of the pioneering work on group dynamics was undertaken some 50 years ago by Kurt Lewin, the German-born American psychologist, and his colleagues whose work led to the view that groups adopt a distinctive personality different from the individual or aggregate characteristics of the individuals who comprise that group. Individuals within groups adopt behavioural patterns and tendencies under the influence of the group whilst at the same time contributing to its identity. These complex interactions are collectively known as group dynamics and were identified as taking place within an environment known as the field-space.

In social psychology, the behaviour of the group can be expressed as a function of personality and environment. Group dynamics have also been described as a four-stage process (Tuckman, 1965). The phases have been identified as:

- forming
- storming

- norming
- performing.

Some observers like to add a fifth element – the mourning!

This developmental model gives a useful insight into dealing with some of the problems of group dynamics and also helps to explain some of the more irrational behaviour that surfaces from time to time.

Although these stages refer to what can be described as the life-cycle of the group over the year, the first four elements also manifest themselves during each of the study day sessions and presenters need to recognise the characteristics.

- *Stage 1* – This stage is characterised by uncertainty, resistance and sometimes suspicion. The VDPs are perhaps testing each other, and the presenter.
- *Stage 2* – The storming phase can be disruptive because there may be evidence of mild aggression arising from frustration, rebellion arising from resistance and challenge arising from uncertainty.
- *Stage 3* – Norming reflects evolving group identity and cohesion amongst the individual members. The features of the earlier stages start to fade and the group begins to show unity and consensus.
- *Stage 4* – This stage is characterised by meaningful achievement and the group starts to work at the task at hand and aims to achieve the desired outcome.
- *Stage 5* – The group begins to disband as the VT year draws to a close.

Leadership

The group will take its behavioural cues from the leader. An effective group leader should be able to:

- promote group autonomy
- protect weaker individuals within the group
- encourage less participative members to contribute to discussion whilst controlling more vociferous individuals
- recognise antagonistic trends
- facilitate the discussions
- monitor, maintain and stimulate performance on an on-going basis
- ensure the discussions remain within the boundaries of the subject matter.

Dealing with difficult situations

Experienced presenters will be only too aware of the 'difficult' group members whose behavioural tendencies can alter group performance. Difficult individuals include those who are reticent or quiet and shy as well as those who are assertive, aggressive and dominant.

Hesitant individuals can be encouraged to participate by pairing group members and inviting each member of the pair to report back after discussion. Hesitancy may reflect lack of confidence and directing 'easy' questions to these individuals can help them overcome shyness.

In contrast, some individuals can dominate group discussions. In a well-balanced group, peer pressure can control this dominance, but this will not happen if other members are subdued or passive. One way of limiting this is to target other individuals to express their views. The clinical experience amongst VDPs can vary enormously as some individuals may have worked in the hospital environment and/or in General Dental Services (GDS) as assistants. They can also dominate discussions because they see themselves as 'the voice of experience' and the group leader should again divert some of the questions to others in the group.

From time to time, *argumentative individuals* can make a presenter's life difficult. Their attitude and argumentative tendencies are often evident in their body language and, whilst contrasting or conflicting opinions can fuel healthy debate, persistent quarrelling can be counter-productive. The best way to deal with this situation is to invite views from the rest of the group – *'Do you agree with that?'* – but avoid confrontation at all costs. Agree and affirm any good points, but do not be led into an argumentative debate on others. If a situation arises where a consensus view cannot be arrived at, it is sometimes better to draw discussions to a close and 'agree to disagree'.

The *non-attentive* or *non-listening* VDP can be dealt with by inviting them to repeat or add their interpretation to a view that has already been expressed by someone else. It may cause initial embarrassment if they haven't been listening, and may alert them sufficiently so that they do not do the same again.

The *political commentator* wants to challenge the system and question its ethics, fairness and values. In this situation, it is best to make a clear statement that you are not empowered to change or influence policy and that your remit is to make the best of the situation that exists.

Getting started

There are numerous teaching methods and lectures and group activities are the most widely used in vocational training.

Lecturing

Didactic lectures have limited value when addressing individual VT schemes, but are useful in situations where a number of schemes have gathered. The main disadvantage of the lecture format is that it discourages participation, but when delivered well can act as a catalyst for further learning.

See Chapter 9 for further information on presentation skills.

Group work

Group work is conducive to participative learning. The VDP group is divided into sub-groups of three or four members and is then set a task. Each sub-group should be asked to elect or nominate a leader, a scribe and a third person who will present their efforts to the main group. This ensures maximum participation of all sub-group members.

Five types of exercise are commonly used in group work activity. These are:

- springboard prompts
- problem solving
- case discussion
- syndication
- role play.

Springboard prompts
Virtually anything can trigger a group discussion, and reference to new materials, controversial techniques, radiographs, etc. can be a springboard for broader discussion. In a planned presentation, the tutor who is leading the session should provide this initial prompt.

Problem solving
This is a challenging and intellectually stimulating exercise that helps the trainees to apply their knowledge and experience to a given situation. Groups should be encouraged to analyse the problem and come up with a variety of solutions and relate these to materials and methods. Tutors

should themselves be thoroughly familiar with alternative solutions so that they are in a position to lead and guide controversial discussions. There is nothing more embarrassing than the trainer who is caught out because he or she is ill prepared.

Case discussion
Case discussion is a valuable group work activity. The cases under discussion should be chosen to illustrate a specific point or act as a prompt to discuss an aspect of treatment planning.

There are four stages to case discussion.

1 The tutor sets the ground rules and lists the objectives.
2 This is a private study period where each individual is given a certain time to think about the case and focus on the objectives outlined in stage 1.
3 The VDPs are divided into sub-groups of three or four to share their thoughts within the privacy of the group and arrive at a consensus view.
4 This is the plenary session where the sub-groups present their conclusions.

Trainers should present the clinical facts in a precise way to ensure that all trainees have the same basic information. Ambiguities lead to different assumptions by different people. This defeats the main aim of the exercise because everyone is looking at the case from a slightly different angle. However, the deliberate introduction of vague information to encourage lateral thinking is permissible, provided that the tutor is sufficiently experienced to handle the diverse outcomes.

Syndication
The syndication process divides an exercise or problem into its component parts; each sub-group is asked to analyse one part of the overall picture. The sub-groups then merge and present the total solution. This technique requires careful advance preparation by the speaker and is only suitable to disciplines that lend themselves to easy division into sub-categories.

Small group teaching is a very rewarding activity for both trainers and VDPs if it is carried out well. The key to success is planning and variety. Research into teaching methods has repeatedly demonstrated the popularity of the small group approach, *see* Box 8.1 and Box 8.2.

Always plan the content of the presentation in advance and prepare the material for group work. The balance between group work and lecturing will be dependent upon the nature of the subject(s) under

Box 8.1 The tutor's perspective on small group teaching

- 'The informal atmosphere provided the opportunity to get to know students at a personal level and for them to get to know me.'
- 'Their attainment is not constrained by pressures of curriculum, difficulties associated with large group inflexibility and above all passive lethargy in a mass lecture environment.'
- 'Feeling of informality and, when things go right, that students have learnt something and, even in statistics, enjoyed themselves.'
- 'Seeing a student suddenly grasp an idea for the first time, which makes, for him, a number of other disjointed areas simultaneously fall into place.'
- 'I can be stimulated by students' ideas.'
- 'Hearing the spontaneous insights of students.'
- 'Opportunity for providing instantaneous, personal feedback on my own thoughts and efforts.'
- 'Being able to give praise.'
- 'The educational goals are readily defined, almost as a contract between myself and the group.'
- 'Talking. Contradicting superficial ideas!'

Box 8.2 The learner's perspective on small group teaching

- 'I personally have a greater influence on what is being discussed. I can actually remember, and feel I understand what we are discussing.'
- 'You can discuss issues together rather than be told them.'
- 'Being able to participate and to find out other people's ideas.'
- 'Being able to discuss and having queries sorted out there and then.'
- 'It is less formal, less intimidating. There is the possibility of asking questions. I think you learn more.'
- 'You get more individual attention.'
- 'I like the flexibility of a small group. We aren't bound to a rigid schedule.'
- 'It teaches you how to converse in a literate manner.'
- 'It helps develop your power of analysing problems and arriving at solutions.'
- 'By being in a smaller group, one feels part of the class rather than just another face in a sea of faces. I actually feel more part of the university.'

discussion. The VT adviser normally provides speakers with a detailed brief on what is expected of them during the session to ensure that presentations are tailored to meet the needs of the group.

Role play

Role-playing is a valuable technique but should be used with caution. The technique can be looked at as an enactment of a real-life situation where the participants can express feelings and views in a non-threatening way. The participants should be given clear and concise information on what is expected of them and should be allowed to prepare for the exercise. The objectives of the role play should be clearly stated, as should the end-point. The exercise may be time-limited or should proceed to a point where there is a natural conclusion. It should be emphasised to the two participants that they are not to take any comments personally and that they should *'step into role'* when the exercise starts and *'step out'* when it concludes. This contains the exercise and avoids exchanges after the role play has finished.

At the end of the role play, ask the rest of the group to complete their observations and invite the participants to do the same.

To be effective role plays should:

- reproduce real-life situations as closely as possible
- develop confidence
- provide an opportunity to practise communication skills
- provide an opportunity to experiment with new approaches
- explore attitudes
- prepare VDPs for encounters that will place them under stress in a real-life situation.

If role plays are not successful it is usually for one of the following reasons:

- overacting
- treating the exercise as futile
- playing it for laughs
- poor briefing on what is expected of the participants.

CHAPTER 9

Presentation skills

Trainers are encouraged to participate as presenters on the study days. Their wealth of experience and expertise gained over many years in general dental practice can support numerous presentations on a variety of topics. Despite this, many shy away from the opportunity for a number of reasons that were alluded to in the last chapter and which fall into one or more of the following categories:

- a reluctance to value their own experience
- concerns about their presentation skills
- uncertainty about what is expected of them.

In other words, concerns that all presenters have at the outset of their presentation careers and many continue to have throughout their careers!

This chapter covers the fundamental principles of presentation skills.

Ten golden rules

1 Define the objective

This may seem like an obvious statement, but it is surprising how many presentations flounder because the speaker has not clearly defined the purpose. It is useful to work to the SMART principle. SMART is an acronym for:

- specific
- measurable
- achievable
- realistic
- timed.

The VT adviser will normally give speakers a brief on the purpose of the presentation and you should ask yourself what you want the VDPs to achieve by the end of the session. There should be a way of measuring this result and the presentation should be structured to allow this to happen. It can happen in a number of ways. In an interactive session, there will be many opportunities for feedback and this will give you a good indication on how effectively you have communicated your message. Another option is to include some practical exercises and group work that will 'test' the group to see whether they can apply the principles that have been discussed. It is important to note that it is not always possible to measure the outcome accurately because behavioural change may not appear until much later when the VDPs are back in their practices.

Avoid the common error of trying to do too much in too little time.

2 Remember your audience

There are a number of audience-related factors, which will affect your presentation. The four main factors are:

- relevance
- sequence
- ownership
- repetition.

The audience must relate to the presentation. The easiest way to achieve this is to put yourself in the shoes of a VDP and try to gain an understanding of their perspective. The key to this is empathy – the ability to see things from another's viewpoint. This will have the effect of engaging the audience from the outset and will enable you to 'take them with you' for the remainder of the presentation. This is particularly important in vocational training where a high level of interaction is desirable.

Sequencing is important in all presentations. There should be a structure to the presentation and the sequence of facts and ideas should be logical and should follow on from one another. This is sometimes referred to as 'forward association', a process that demonstrates that people remember things in the order in which they are communicated.

It is also helpful to know who is in the group, what the range of experience is amongst the group members and what subjects have been covered in the study days. Groups will be more interactive after the first few weeks when group identity has been established (*see* Chapter 8 on small group teaching).

One of the most common mistakes is to take a presentation you may have given to a different audience and then repeat it in the same way to a group of VDPs. This rarely works, although it may do for a very limited range of subjects. Presentations should be adapted to suit the audience.

3 Use a variety of audio-visual aids

The choice of audio-visual aids will depend on the type of information you want to convey, the size of the audience, the arrangement of the room and the AV facilities available. If you have been invited to give a presentation, you will normally be asked for a list of your requirements.

The visual aids most commonly used are:

- flipcharts
- overhead projectors (OHPs)
- 35-mm slides
- video
- computer-generated presentations
- whiteboards
- handouts.

The best way to learn about the use of different audio-visual aids is to observe experienced presenters – after all they have all learnt the same way!

Flipcharts are always useful in any interactive presentation and have the advantage that they offer a visual record of spontaneity – the audio-visual aid develops as the presentation goes along. They can be useful for recording the outcome of group work or setting/writing down objectives at the outset of the presentation. Some pages can be prepared in advance and it is also easy to look back at previous pages of work. The main disadvantage is that they are not portable and can look messy if used carelessly.

Flipcharts charts can be used more effectively if you:

- tear off pages and post them to the wall
- use different coloured felt pens and remember to check that the felt pens work *before* you start – it is surprising how many pens have dried out during a presentation!
- try and use symbols and diagrams rather than just words.

Overhead projectors are readily available in all postgraduate centres. They can be used in bright lighting conditions and can be used with prepared material or for spontaneous jottings down. Their main disadvantage is that there is a limit to how much information can be legibly projected and many inexperienced presenters make the mistake of cramming too much information onto a single overhead acetate sheet. (A useful rule of thumb is to keep to no more than six lines per page and maintain a 6 mm minimum height on the lettering for predictable projection.)

The projection lens can also obstruct the view of the screen, particularly in a small group setting, although this could be avoided by changing the seating arrangements in advance of the presentation.

The transparency itself (sometimes called an acetate or foil) can be produced in a number of ways. It can be printed directly from a laser or inkjet printer, but you must select the correct type of acetate. Acetates for laser printers are different from those for inkjet printers. Inkjet acetates are coated on one side to 'hold' the ink. There is usually a marker on the sheet to tell you which side is coated. Photocopying from a paper copy is another method, but make sure that the acetates are photocopier compatible.

Useful ideas for using OHPs are as follows:

• if you want to reveal the information progressively, then a plain piece of paper can be used to cover the hidden element – thin paper is as effective as thick paper but has the advantage that the presenter can see through it and read the obscured text
• use a pen or pencil on the projector as a pointer. This is better than pointing to something on the screen
• using overlays can help to construct more complex images.

The 35-mm slide format has stood the test of time in postgraduate education. Slides can be used in single, double or triple projection techniques, but most postgraduate centres restrict double and triple projection facilities to the lecture theatre and these techniques are therefore better suited to a larger audience, but may be used in clinical presentations to illustrate cases and techniques. The main disadvantage is that the room may need to be 'blacked out' and the presenter loses eye contact with the audience. Slides take time to produce and can be costly. They cannot be updated, only reproduced with the changes incorporated.

Here are some helpful tips for using slides:

• keep to one idea/concept per slide
• label your slide mounts and mark them in one corner so they can be inserted correctly into the carousel. This marking is called a thumb spot and is usually placed on the lower left-hand corner of each slide. Slides are then inserted upside down in the carousel so that all the thumb

spots are visible on the top right-hand corner. A glance at your carousel will show you that you have them the right way round
- always have a test run to preview your slides to make sure they are in the right order and the right way up
- look at your audience and not at your slide
- use blanks or scenic slides as a break between two parts of a presentation
- do not overdo the number of slides you have. Twenty-five slides are often sufficient for a one-hour presentation – unless you have a number that build up a number of bullet points
- keep to six lines per slide and six words per line
- avoid mixing landscape and portrait formats
- try to combine graphics and words in the design
- use a laser pointer to draw attention to specific areas on your slide, but do not overuse it. It is particularly useful if you want to draw attention to a specific aspect of an image but would not be needed if you were using bullet points to highlight text
- use a remote control so that you can move around the room
- if you are using dual projection check how the remote control operates. A single control will advance both projectors, but you will need separate controls if you want to advance one independently of the other.

Playback video is a very useful tool and gives the audience moving images, which can be a welcome break from static images, but it should be used only when it serves to illustrate a point or stimulate discussion.
Things to bear in mind include:

- the tape should be 'cued' so that it is 'ready to roll' at the moment it is needed
- check the volume and ensure that it is appropriate for the seating arrangements and the setting
- use a remote control so that you can pause the tape for discussion and interaction.

Increasingly, many presenters are now turning to computers to create their presentations. A presentation package offers many advantages, not least of which is the ease with which changes can be made to update material. Many presentation packages offer a number of design features, which include picture effects, sound, transitions and a host of text effects. These should be used sparingly because an audience soon tires of 'gimmicks', which can detract from the message.
The basic rules are:

- be professional in appearance and design
- produce uncluttered material with an easy to read font
- restrict key points to no more than six per slide
- do not use a font size smaller than 16–18 points
- avoid using all upper case letters
- refrain from too many gimmicks.

4 Produce support material

This is commonly in the form of handouts and it is always the presenter's dilemma to decide at what stage the handouts should be made available. If they are distributed at the beginning of the presentation, the advantage is that group members can follow the presentation on the handout and supplement the information recorded with additional notes. The disadvantage is that the handout tends to give away the sequencing of the presentation and it is difficult for members of a group to resist the temptation to flick ahead to the next section before the presenter wants them to. If the handouts are given at the end, then the group will not have had the benefit of adding to them but will rely on notes they may have made on separate pieces of paper and the two sets will then have to be collated.

The decision rests with the individual and to some extent depends on the nature of the presentation. If there are lists of resources and facts that are discussed, then these can be made available at the end and in summary form.

5 Consider room layout and seating arrangements

The seating arrangements should be conducive to interaction and should allow all individuals equal access to view any visuals. The arrangements will be limited to the room size. *See* Chapter 8 for a review of different seating positions.

6 Style and substance

There is no doubt that an audience values style of presentation as much as it does the substance. Remember to be yourself and deliver the presentation in a style and manner compatible with your personality. It takes time to create your own brand of presentation. It is a good idea to observe other presenters and see how they combine style and substance elements in their presentation. Although it is tempting to copy a successful presentation style this rarely works because sooner or later the incompatibility of your personality and someone's else style will come through and will be detrimental to the perception the audience has of you.

The content of your presentation should have a general dental practice focus, unless you have been asked specifically to speak about issues outside general practice.

Most presentations in vocational training are given to small groups of 10–12 people. This group size is ideal for interactive presentations and so try and involve your audience at all times. Part of your presentation may need to be didactic and formal to lead the group into a scene where discussion and interaction predominate, but take care to plan for some interaction at some stage in the presentation.

7 Catch the attention of your audience

This is essential from the outset when you most need to engage the audience. The audience will make a value judgement on your presentation in the first few minutes and it is important that you grab their attention quickly. Some presenters will use humorous anecdotes, some rely on deliberate provocation, particularly when controversial issues are to be discussed, and others start with questions.

Try to tell the audience a story, but make it have some relevance to the subject of the presentation. Examples of incidents and events from your own personal and professional experience will give an additional dimension to your presentation. This is one of the oldest rhetoric devices in history and has been used by some of the world's greatest orators. Not only will it make your presentation more interesting, but the device has lasting educational value because your audience will be more likely to remember the lessons from a good tale than they will from a list of bullet points from a textbook.

8 Be confident

Like many skills, the secret of success is practice. A leading novel writer was famously asked the secret of good writing, to which he replied 'rewriting'. One of the world's leading violinists was asked how he managed to play the violin so well, to which he replied 'by playing the violin'. If you want to become a good speaker, the only way is to speak and speak often.

You are in charge of your audience. Their thoughts, emotions and perceptions are under your control and a good presenter will engage with the audience from the very start. The way you dress, speak and interact will influence this perception. The relative positioning of the presenter within the group is very important in a small group setting – less so in didactic lecturing where the presenter is expected to be centre stage or behind a podium. Remember to pay attention to your body language – your audience can read a lot into how you stand or sit or the way you walk!

Never begin your presentation by apologising for your nervousness – appear confident and in control at all times. One way of overcoming nervousness is to meet your audience before you begin. Arrive at the centre early and join the VDPs for their morning coffee or over the lunch break. Not only will it help you to get to know your audience, but it also helps to overcome nerves. Remember that some nervousness is an asset as it can enhance your presentation.

The VT adviser normally gives the group a summary of your career to date. This is a good way of earning respect from the outset.

(It is a good idea to summarise the highlights of your career in bullet points and bring it with you on the day or send it to the VT adviser in advance. Not only does this look professional but it also shows that you are organised.)

9 Review your material

There is no such thing as the perfect presentation. Improvements can always be made. It is a good idea to review the structure of your planned presentation a few days after you have undertaken the planning process and revise the format. It is surprising how something can seem like a great idea one day but appears lacklustre a few days later.

10 Rehearse

As the 19th-century essayist William Hazlitt wrote 'We never do anything well till we cease to think about the manner of doing it'. The key to a successful presentation is rehearsal. Rehearsal will make you familiar with the substance of your presentation to such an extent that you will not need to think about content when you perform in front of the group. This leaves you free to focus on interacting with the audience on the day.

Structure

At a basic level, all presentations should be planned in three sections: the beginning, middle and end.

The introduction should give the audience a very clear indication of what you intend to cover during the presentation. It should also set the tone and style of the presentation and give the audience an indication of what you expect from them. You can use the introduction to set the ground rules for your presentation by outlining, for example, when you want to take questions and how you intend to run the session.

The middle of the presentation will contain the relevant facts, data, references and opinions relating to the subject matter under consideration. The material in this section should be carefully organised and arranged to ensure that there is a continuity of thought during this phase of the presentation.

The end should contain the key points from the core of the presentation; it is always a good idea to relate these to your introduction. This helps the audience to fit everything together and is a good way to conclude the presentation. You may wish to finish with an anecdote, a question or some ideas for the group to think about, but remember that a snappy ending has as much impact as a snappy opening.

Another structure, proposed by Brown, identifies four features that optimise clarity during presentations (Brown, 1982). These are:

1 *Signposts* – Signposts tell the group the direction you will be taking. Statements such as 'Today I propose to discuss four aspects of practice management. The first is ...'
2 *Frames* – The frame helps to delineate sections of a presentation. Statements such as 'Now, we are going to look at the medico-legal aspects of endodontics ...'
3 *Foci* – Foci are statements that highlight and emphasise key facts. For example, 'The common causes of instrument separation in endodontics are ...'
4 *Links* – Links are used to maintain continuity between the different sections of the presentation. They help the flow of the presentation. Links can be added by statements but can also be included by using visual images.

Seven rules for success

1 Use names

If you are asked to give a presentation to a VT group, you are likely to spend the entire session with them, or in some cases the whole day. One effective way to gain their trust, approval and confidence is to remember their names. It will make the question-and-answer sessions more personal and it will allow you to selectively ask individuals their views on certain things if you have realised that they have some expertise in a particular area. It will also make the session more intimate and friendly.

Many people find it difficult to remember names. Here are some tips from experienced speakers on how to remember names.

- When you hear someone's name repeat it in your mind at least three times whilst looking at them. Try to form an association between the name and the face (the more absurd the association, the easier it will be to recall the name and you need not worry because you do not have to divulge the association!).
- Some speakers find it is a useful technique to imagine the name written on the person's forehead.
- Repeat the name back to the individual when they tell you.

2 Control your audience

This is an important skill because if you do not control the group, you will risk losing your way during the presentation. Audiences are expert at distracting their speakers and you must be disciplined enough to control them without appearing to do so. Here are some ways that you can do this

- *Move around the room* – the distraction keeps the audience alert and it means that the sound of your voice hits them from different angles. It also helps to engage all members of the group because you will be nearer to some than others at different points during your movement. If you are using audio-visual aids without a remote device, for example, an OHP, return to the projector in good time to change the image.
- *Stop talking* and *seek views* from the group to confirm their understanding of what you have said.
- After a break, groups can sometimes start to chat and it can be difficult to attract their attention. Simply *assume your speaking pose and remain silent.* Your body language will tell them you want to start and the ambient chatter will soon die down.

If you make a mistake, do not panic. It happens to the best presenters. Do not put yourself down in front of the audience. Accept what has happened with dignity and without embarrassment.

If you are worried about forgetting your lines, then don't; you should not be memorising your presentation anyway.

If there is a technical breakdown, acknowledge it and carry on. It is a mistake to pretend it never happened.

3 Be yourself

Your style of presentation should be a reflection of your personality. There may be similarities between the stage actor and the speaker, but it does not go as far as trying to be someone else.

4 Interact with your audience

Interaction with the audience is more than just inviting them to participate verbally. A variety of non-verbal skills should be used because participants will pick up messages from your posture, hand movements, facial gestures and eye contact. When you make eye contact with members of your audience, hold your gaze for a few seconds – just long enough to engage them without intimidating them. Remember that you are getting feedback from their body language as much as they are from yours.

Inviting questions plays an important part in an interactive session. Inexperienced presenters (and experienced ones for that matter) often worry about how to deal with questions. Here are some tips.

- Repeat or paraphrase the question so that the audience knows what is being asked – this also helps you to be sure what you have been asked. It also buys those extra few precious seconds for your brain to formulate the answer.
- Always remain courteous and polite no matter how aggressive the question.
- If you do not know the answer, then say so, but say also you will endeavour to find out or invite the audience to answer.

5 Become part of your audience

Talk to them as colleagues, not as outsiders – you will earn more respect. In the 1980s, the concept of Management by Walking Around (MBWA) was put forward by Peters and Waterman in their book *In Search of Excellence* (Peters and Waterman, 1988). They talked about managers and workers working alongside one another to implement change. You can apply the same principle, because it is true of the presenter and the audience.

If your natural presentation style is informal, try sitting with the group rather than standing. If they are seated, this will make you part of them.

6 Use personal experiences and stories

There is nothing an audience likes more than to hear real-life examples from your own experience. These stories are the flesh and blood on the skeleton, which is the structure of your presentation.

7 Pace your presentation

Vary the pace of your delivery and the tone of your voice. Use silence, pauses and images on your slides to close one train of thought and start another. Remember the French proverb, 'The spoken word belongs half to the one who speaks it and half to the one who hears it'. Always try to engage with your audience.

Feedback

There will be an evaluation of your presentation by the VDPs at the end, and a copy of the summary is available for the speaker. There are many variations of evaluation forms in use throughout the country. They are constantly changing in an effort to make them yield useful and relevant information.

Not only will the VDPs be asked to evaluate your session using one of a variety of forms, but also you will be asked to give feedback on your involvement to complete the loop.

The evaluation summary is very important because it helps you to evolve as a presenter. Do not be unduly upset if there is criticism and do not get carried away with their adulation of your style. Remember what they say in the Hollywood movie industry – the secret of lasting success is not to believe your own publicity!

CHAPTER 10

Assessment

Assessment has been defined as 'the process of measuring the learner's acquisition of cognitive, effective and psychomotor skills'. Its primary purpose is to find out where the VDP is at any given stage in their training. It is given a high priority in dental vocational training because it provides essential information to set short, medium and long-term training goals. Sometimes the terms 'assessment', 'appraisal' and 'evaluation' are used interchangeably but they all have very specific meanings in the educational sense. Appraisal is a process of 'regular meetings between teacher and learner with support for the benefit of the learner'. It is a non-threatening and friendly approach and reflects the principles of formative assessment (discussed later in this chapter) (*see also* Chapter 4). Evaluation is the process of 'measuring the teaching'.

The purposes of assessment are to:

- identify the needs of the VDP
- plan the in-practice training programme
- monitor VDP progress
- diagnose problems – sometimes referred to as diagnostic assessment
- adjust the pace of the learning
- judge the effectiveness of training
- assess trainer effectiveness.

In general, if assessment is to provide useful information it must:

- be objective and analytical
- lead to constructive comments
- take place at regular intervals and on a continual basis
- involve both parties
- form the basis of the future development of the training programme.

These principles can be applied to a range of circumstances both in the practice and on the VT study course.

Timing

It is not uncommon for trainers and VDPs to outline learning objectives in the early weeks of the training year and then base the bulk of training on an initial diagnostic assessment.

Box 10.1 Clinical experience checklist

Please use the key to help you complete the checklist and tick the appropriate column. Add any other comments that you feel would help you to plan the next few weeks with your trainer.

Key
0 no opportunity to learn
1 little opportunity to practise
2 several opportunities to practise
3 considerable experience

Week 1 date: ....

| | *Key* | | | | |
	0	1	2	3	*Comments*
Diagnosis					
Radiology					
Treatment planning					
Prescribing					
Control of pain					
Paedodontics					
Orthodontics					
Prevention					
Periodontics					
Conservation					
Endodontics					
Crown and bridgework					
Oral surgery					
Oral medicine					
Prosthodontics					
Treatment involving GA/sedation					
Dental emergencies: toothache/trauma					
Knowledge of medical emergencies					
CPR training					Date of last practice:

The initial training agreement and clinical experience checklist, *see* Box 10.1, are essential parts of the professional development portfolio. They give the VDP and the trainer an opportunity to share information that will enhance and support the training programme.

In the early part of the year reassessment should take place at weekly intervals. This time span may then be increased to monthly reviews for the remainder of the year. These time intervals are not set in tablets of stone, as much will depend on the VDP's learning style and on the number of training opportunities that arise during the early months. The key features of continuous assessment are that:

• it takes place during the training process in everyday practising conditions
• it allows trainers to use a planned tutorial to assess achievement and progress
• it is transparent and makes VDPs continually aware of the criteria against which they are assessed
• it encourages the regular use of the professional development portfolio to track progress and experience.

Three useful resources that contribute to this are to be found in the portfolio. They are:

1 *professional development log* – this is essentially a reflective tool (*see* Box 10.2)
2 *practice activity log* – this is a statistical review of progress and relates workload to the financial aspects of dentistry
3 *work analysis log* – first introduced in 1990, then incorporated in the original VT Record Book (*see* Box 10.3).

Other on-going opportunities may trigger the need for assessment, for example:

• whenever the trainer feels that the VDP can demonstrate progress
• when the trainer wants to know if progress is being made – perhaps in a particular aspect of care that may have been the subject of hands-on help or a tutorial
• when process skills need to be assessed, e.g. problem solving
• in the event of a significant occurrence which has triggered an incident.

Assessment methods

The selection of methodology should reflect certain criteria, which include:

• *purpose* – how will the findings be used?

Box 10.2 Professional development weekly log

Week 3 starting: ....

Please think back over the past week and make
some notes to help you reflect on your experience,
and plan your future activities. You can use this log
to help identify issues for discussion in your weekly
tutorial sessions.

Achievements:

Concerns:

Incident analysis:
what happened?

what are your thoughts now?

what have you learned from the analysis?

Action plan:

Box 10.3 Work analysis log

	Date	Date	Date	Date	Date
DIAGNOSIS					
Extensive exam					
Radiographs					
Study models					
RESTORATIVE					
Crown (Ant)					
Crown (Post)					
Cast post					
Conventional bridge					
Adhesive bridge					
Veneer					
Pin retention					
Posterior composite					
ENDODONTICS					
RCT (anterior)					
RCT (premolar)					
RCT (molar)					
PROSTHODONTICS					
F/F					
Partial (acrylic)					
Partial (Co-Cr)					
ORAL SURGERY					
XLA-simple					
XLA-orthodontic					
Surgical-soft tissue					
Surgical-bone removal					
Apicectomy					
PERIODONTICS					
Visit 1: scaling					
Visit 2: scaling					
Full mouth perio					
ORTHODONTICS					
Case assessment					
Removable appliances					
MISCELLANEOUS					
Acute pain control					
Trauma					
Referral letters					
Rubber dam					
Domiciliary visits					
Emergency call out					
Mouth guards: sports					
RCT (deciduous)					
SPECIAL INTERESTS/ OWN TOPICS					

- *impact* – how will these findings impact on training activity?
- *validity* – does it measure what it set out to measure?
- *fairness* – does it allow the VDPs to demonstrate what they know?
- *reliability* – is the information reliable enough to allow trainers to compare it with other trainers on the scheme or with previous VDPs?
- *significance* – does the process address the content and skills that relate to current clinical practice?
- *efficiency* – is the assessment method time-efficient in relation to other activities?

The use of assessment tools should be seen as positive and non-threatening. It should not degenerate into opportunistic or outright criticism and the outcomes should remain confidential to the parties involved.

Assessment protocols should be used to elicit information from a number of different perspectives. These can be conveniently grouped under the specific categories of:

- *declarative knowledge* – the *'what'* knowledge
- *conditional knowledge* – the *'why'* knowledge
- *procedural knowledge* – the *'how'* knowledge
- *application knowledge* – the *'use'* of knowledge in different contexts
- *problem solving* – the use of knowledge and/or skills to resolve a situation
- *critical thinking* – the evaluation of concepts associated with inquiry
- *understanding* – the synthesis by the learner of concepts, processes and skills.

This breakdown will help trainers to plan training requirements objectively because the processes that lead to an improvement in, say, *procedural knowledge* are very different from those designed to enhance *understanding*.

The professional development portfolio

The professional development portfolio (PDP) has superceded the old-style VT Record Book that was an early attempt at recording and monitoring VDP progress. The integration of vocational training with continuing professional development has been the driving force behind its redesign.

It reflects the shift towards outcome-based assessments in postgraduate education rather than the traditional view of 'passing' or 'failing'. This process of on-going monitoring of VDP performance has the following features:

- it takes place during the learning process
- it takes place in real-life everyday conditions
- it is used to help the learner and the learning process (formative)
- it enables trainers to use any planned learning experience (in tutorials, for example) to assess achievements and progress.

These important features are all incorporated in the PDP. It is arranged in four parts, the contents of which are shown in Box 10.4.

Part 1 brings together some baseline information and helps trainers and VDPs set the training agenda. The clinical experience checklist is a useful discussion aid in the early weeks of the training year and helps both parties to record some baseline information relating to clinical experience.

Part 2 is made up of weekly logs, which culminate in a professional development summary, an opportunity to revise the clinical experience

---

Box 10.4 Contents of the professional development portfolio

Introduction

Part 1   **You and the scheme**
Trainer's details
Personal details
Aims and objectives of vocational training
Obligations of trainers and VDPs
Vocational training assessment

Part 2   **Professional development records**
Section 1   *Initial training agreement*
Section 2   *Professional development weekly logs*
Self-assessment 1
Self-assessment 2
Section 3   *Professional development monthly logs*
Self-assessment 3

Part 3   **Final appraisal statements**

Part 4   **Appendices**
1 *Practice activity log*
2 *Work analysis log*
3 *Record of other meetings and courses attended*
4 *Record of clinical attachments undertaken*
5 *Framework for optional analysis of patient activity*
6 *Useful addresses and telephone numbers*
7 *Tutorials log*
Spare weekly/fortnightly logs

checklist in light of the early weeks of practice experience and formulate an action plan for the next phase of training. There are further self-assessments in this section and summary information is recorded in the profile review summary as shown in Box 10.5. Separate and individual assessment allows both parties to score independently, and then to compare the outcomes. If there are significant differences of opinion, it may be necessary to return to first principles and define what are considered to be acceptable standards. Joint assessment should then take place to ensure that consistent criteria are being applied to the procedure.

Part 3 contains the final appraisal statements and *Part 4* contains a selection of useful appendices, to enable VDPs to record additional postgraduate activities, tutorial subjects and analyse their clinical work.

At the end of the training year, the final appraisal statements are completed. This appraisal is in three parts. One part is completed by the VDP, the trainer completes one and the final joint appraisal statement is agreed and signed by both parties. The VT adviser makes a separate adviser's final summary. The postgraduate dental dean retains copies of the latter two documents.

It should be noted that the portfolio remains the property of the VDP and the information contained in it remains confidential to the VDP, the trainer and, for formative assessment purposes, to the adviser and the dean.

Types of assessment

The current debate on this subject centres on concerns about appropriate forms of assessment during the VT year. At the time of writing, VDPs receive a certificate of completion of VT on the basis of contractual adherence. The concerns are that this award does not include a review of performance, but merely reflects the fulfilment of a contractual requirement (Editorial, 1999).

The measurement of progress and performance review has always generated widespread debate in educational circles. There are inherent flaws in any system that tries to measure the quality of clinical performance, but there are nevertheless some ways of achieving this. These include:

- achievement/proficiency assessment
- norm-referencing/criterion referencing
- continuous assessment/fixed-point assessment
- summative assessment/formative assessment
- direct assessment/indirect assessment

Box 10.5 The profile review

Key:

0 no opportunity to practise
1 little experience of this aspect
2 regularly in need of advice
3 need advice occasionally
4 progressing well
5 attaining exceptional standards

Self-management

	0	1	2	3	4	5
I can organise, plan and manage time efficiently	☐	☐	☐	☐	☐	☐
I take initiatives to identify my learning goals	☐	☐	☐	☐	☐	☐
I keep my portfolio and records up to date	☐	☐	☐	☐	☐	☐
I am able to handle the workload	☐	☐	☐	☐	☐	☐

Professional values/interpersonal skills

	0	1	2	3	4	5
I place patient care above all personal considerations	☐	☐	☐	☐	☐	☐
I participate in on-going professional development	☐	☐	☐	☐	☐	☐
I work well as a team member	☐	☐	☐	☐	☐	☐
I am a good communicator and listener	☐	☐	☐	☐	☐	☐
I give patients confidence and relieve anxiety	☐	☐	☐	☐	☐	☐
I am able to make use of and participate in my professional development profile	☐	☐	☐	☐	☐	☐
I have a working knowledge of medico-legal issues such as confidentiality and consent	☐	☐	☐	☐	☐	☐

Clinical

	0	1	2	3	4	5
I have a reasonable knowledge of all appropriate aspects of clinical dentistry so far	☐	☐	☐	☐	☐	☐
I have reasonable knowledge of diagnosis, treatment planning and prognosis	☐	☐	☐	☐	☐	☐
I can deal with dental emergencies effectively	☐	☐	☐	☐	☐	☐
I can routinely work with close support, 4-handed techniques	☐	☐	☐	☐	☐	☐

Administration and management

	0	1	2	3	4	5
I have a working knowledge of:						
a) NHS administrative procedures	☐	☐	☐	☐	☐	☐
b) practice administration procedures	☐	☐	☐	☐	☐	☐
c) basic terms and conditions of the general dental services	☐	☐	☐	☐	☐	☐
I have experience of/participated in appropriate practice management issues	☐	☐	☐	☐	☐	☐
I am able to make appropriate referrals	☐	☐	☐	☐	☐	☐
I can understand and apply the principles of audit reasonably (e.g. analysis of practice activity log)	☐	☐	☐	☐	☐	☐
I have a working knowledge of health and safety legislation (e.g. COSHH, RIDDOR, fire regulations)	☐	☐	☐	☐	☐	☐

VDP:
(signature)
Date:

Trainer:
(signature)
Date:

- subjective assessment/objective assessment
- checklist rating/performance rating
- impression/guided judgement
- holistic assessment/analytic assessment
- assessment by others/self-assessment.

Achievement/proficiency assessment

Achievement assessment is course-orientated and relates to the taught course, whereas proficiency assessment relates to what someone can do in the real world. Traditional teaching leans towards achievement assessment.

Norm-referencing/criterion referencing

Norm referencing refers to the placing of learners in rank order in relation to their peers. It is typical of classroom ranking where someone comes first and someone comes last. Criterion referencing is the assessment of the learner in terms of his or her ability in a particular subject, irrespective of the performance of the other members of the peer group.

Continuous assessment/fixed-point assessment

Continuous assessment takes place throughout the year in contrast to fixed-point assessment, which is a snapshot of performance at a particular time. The examination is a typical example and there are many dental professionals whose competence was never in doubt during their undergraduate training, but who, for whatever reason, failed to perform at a given point in time during a critical examination. Fixed-point assessment has its merits because it can test knowledge, but it does favour a certain type of learner. Continuous assessment in the form of the presentation of a portfolio of work or case reports is generally regarded to be a more appropriate approach in postgraduate education, whereas fixed-point assessment still predominates in many undergraduate institutions.

Summative assessment/formative assessment

Summative assessment is designed to 'sum-up' what the learner can and cannot do at a particular moment in time. It is a 'gateway' approach to education and has dominated undergraduate teaching for a very long time, although there are early signs that this is gradually changing. Those who were able to get through the gate 'passed' and those who did not had 'failed' and repeated failure often led to expulsion from the course. It is a judgemental process and a controversial one in adult education.

There is no summative assessment in dental vocational training. There have been many debates amongst those involved in vocational training about whether some form of end-point assessment should now be introduced to formalise the role of VT in professional development. It is a debate that will gain momentum given the current wave of accountability and governance that is forcing change at all levels. For this reason, it is interesting to make comparisons with the medical profession.

In medicine, summative assessment is used to test a set of competencies that are laid down in the Parliamentary Regulations for General Practice (The NHS (Vocational Training for General Medical Practice) Regulations, 1997). These competencies are identified as:

- factual medical knowledge sufficient to enable the practitioner to perform the duties of a general practitioner
- the ability to apply factual medical knowledge to the management of problems presented by patients in general practice
- effective communication, both orally and in writing
- the ability to consult satisfactorily with general practice patients
- the ability to review and critically analyse the practitioner's own working practices and manage any necessary changes appropriately
- the ability to synthesise all of the above competencies and apply them appropriately in a general practice setting.

The components of summative assessment are:

- multiple choice questionnaire
- trainer's report
- written submission of practical work (at present and audit project)
- assessment of consultation skills (using video).

Although there are no plans to introduce summative assessment in dental vocational training, it cannot be ruled out in the future.

Formative assessment is a continuous process during which the VDP and trainer interact to identify learning needs and then develop strategies to satisfy these needs. There are no performance 'grades' and there is no 'pass' or 'fail'. It is criterion-referenced assessment that measures the performance against the learning criteria in the training programme. In contrast, norm-based assessment measures learners against each other and ranks them in relation to their peers. A lot of summative assessment is norm-based.

If the ultimate purpose of assessment is to support high quality learning, then formative assessment should be perceived as the most important form. In their book *Inside the Black Box*, Black and William make a strong case for formative assessment and stress that learners must be able to self-assess. The authors state that learners should 'understand the main purposes of their learning and thereby grasp what they need to do to achieve'. This perspective is one of the fundamental tenets of dental vocational training. The learner, they argue, is the 'ultimate-user' of the information that formative assessment provides (Black and William, 1998).

The formative assessment cycle is shown in Figure 10.1.

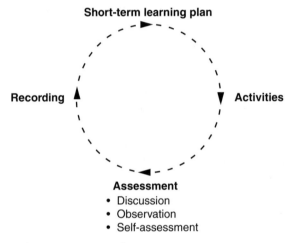

Figure 10.1 Formative assessment cycle.

Direct assessment/indirect assessment

Direct assessment takes place by assessing the learner's performance. For example, a trainer may sit in during a treatment session where the VDP is undertaking a particular procedure. The trainer can observe what the VDP is actually doing and compare it with pre-set criteria (in the form of a grid, for example) and then provide an assessment. In contrast, indirect assessment will usually test the application prowess of the VDP on paper.

Subjective assessment/objective assessment

Subjective assessment is related to observer judgement, whereas objective assessment eliminates the 'judgement' factor and relies on correctness. A multiple-choice question, for example, may have only one right answer and is therefore an excellent objective measure. Objective measures make for meaningful comparisons, whereas bias and personal value judgements influence subjective assessment. Subjectivity can be reduced by providing detailed specifications, pooling judgements from a number of people so that no one person's bias can totally influence outcome and also by weighting different factors.

Checklist rating/performance rating

A scale rating places an individual at a level within a framework that comprises a number of different levels. It is based on a 'ladder principle' and the assessor places the individual on a particular rung. Each rung has a definition associated with it, or the definition may be broad, identifying only the bottom, middle and top of the structure. The checklist rating is simply a list where the assessor ticks the presence or absence of whatever is on the list. A health and safety check during a VT practice visit is one example.

Impression/guided judgement

Impression assessment is totally subjective and is made on the basis of experience. The process can be made more objective by reducing the subjectivity by a commitment to assess against given criteria. Patients will often assess the VDP on the basis of subjective impressions. For example, a particularly youthful-looking VDP is not perceived to be a real dentist! If the VDP then carries out a procedure he or she is supplying the patient with objective measures, such as absence of pain during the administration of anaesthesia, or the relief of pain after the procedure or an observable improvement in aesthetics, which allows for a more objective assessment.

Holistic assessment/analytic assessment

Holistic assessment, as the term suggests, relates to taking an overall, all-embracing perspective on performance rather than breaking down performance into individual components.

Assessment by others/self-assessment

Assessment by others may involve the trainer, the VT adviser, the post-graduate dean and the patient, whereas self-assessment focuses on judgements about the VDP's own proficiency. The main advantage of self-assessment is that it is a motivational aid to the VDP and helps them to recognise their own strengths and weaknesses and learning needs. It is one of the tenets of vocational training. Given the current concerns about measuring the 'success' of the VT year, it seems likely that outside assessment will play an increasing part in the future of training programmes and that trainers may well be required to play a key role in this.

Common errors

Unless experienced, trainers and VDPs can fall victim to what is described as the 'halo effect' and the 'horn effect'.

The *'halo effect'* refers to a tendency to see someone through rose-coloured spectacles. The reasons for this effect can be one or more on any of the following:

* *compatibility* – it is easy to show positive bias toward someone who has pleasant manners and always agrees with your own way of thinking
* *immediacy* – if someone has performed exceptionally well at a given moment or period in time, this observation is immediately allowed to displace their mediocrity of under-performance at a previous time
* *the no-complaints scenario* – if the VDP has no complaints to discuss, the erroneous assumption is made that everything must be satisfactory.

The 'horn effect' describes a tendency to give someone a lower assessment than the true circumstances justify. Some possible causes for this are:

* the trainer is a perfectionist and is unwilling to give credit to less than perfect outcomes
* the trainer disagrees with the VDP or has a different set of values – this may exert a negative bias on VDP performance
* the dramatic incident effect allows a recent mistake to wipe out all previous achievements
* the personality trait effect, where a VDP who may be brash, weak or passive (or is lacking in any particular personality trait which the trainer holds in high regard) may receive a lower rating than is actually warranted

• the different approach effect, which relates to underscoring performance because someone has approached a problem from an angle different from the one the trainer was expecting, even though the outcome may be totally satisfactory.

The value of joint assessment should help to eliminate some of this bias, and trainers and VDPs should discuss significant differences in their perceptions of progress to ascertain if any of the above have influenced the outcome.

Acting on results

The feedback mechanism is an essential prerequisite for professional development. It only works when the VDP is in a position to notice, record and interpret events and situations. Interpretation, in particular, requires sufficient pre-knowledge and understanding if the VDP is expected to identify learning needs arising from an 'adverse' incident. The principles of effective feedback are:

• *allow the VDP to speak first* – ask the question 'how did you feel it went?'
• *always deal with the positive aspects before the negative aspects*
• *turn negatives into positives* – if that didn't work too well, what else could you have done? What might you do next time?
• *be specific with feedback* – 'I noticed that you' . . . NOT 'you were terrible!'.

Practice-based training should be outcome-based. Ultimately, however assessment is carried out and whatever tools are used it is the impact of the information that will affect VDP performance and progress. Nobody expects trainers to turn their VDPs into master clinicians who can claim to have perfected all competencies.

There has been much research into the development of an assessment system for dental vocational training. It has been suggested that a formal assessment process is needed to ensure that the educational objectives are met, and that the use of competency statements, such as 'the VDP can demonstrate to an appropriate standard the ability to manage difficult patients', may be one way of defining an acceptable level of competence (Prescott *et al.*, 2001).

CHAPTER 11

The study days

The VT study course provides the formal educational component of vocational training and is designed to complement in-practice training opportunities. Most study days are held at a suitable postgraduate centre within the regional boundaries of the postgraduate deanery. Occasionally, some courses may be held elsewhere to take advantage of particular facilities that are not available at the centre.

Course design

VDPs are required to attend 30 study days, normally scheduled once a week over three 10-week terms. The VT adviser selects the duration of each term and the term dates, normally at the beginning of each year. In recent years there have been many variations on the three 10-week term format. For example, some trainers have advocated a 'front-loading' approach to the course in which over half the annual study days are condensed into the first term. The thinking behind this change has been to better prepare the VDPs for the remainder of the year. In some cases this can mean having as many as 15–20 study days in the first term, which then leaves fewer days to accommodate over the remaining months of the year.

The idea has not met with universal approval amongst VDPs; whilst they welcome the initiative in some ways, they frequently complain that they lose touch with their peer group during the latter part of the year as there are fewer opportunities to meet in the formal setting of a study day. This observation in itself reflects the value they place on peer group support.

Inevitably, there will be some regional variation on the precise duration of each term depending on the course content. For example, a residential course will involve an overnight stay and trainers would be expected to release their trainee from the practice for the additional day. The remainder of the term dates will normally be adjusted to compensate for any extra days.

Trainers are expected to encourage regular and punctual attendance of their VDP on the study days and are welcome to attend any of the sessions by prior arrangement with the VT adviser. Trainers are expected to monitor and supervise the VDP's attendance on the course and to ensure that holidays are taken outside term time. It is a requirement of the course that VDPs make up any missed sessions in their own time.

The study days

The purpose of the study days is to provide an opportunity for formal teaching on all aspects of general dental practice. In addition, the study course provides opportunities for:

• peer discussion
• exposure to a variety of presenters
• learning from the experience of others
• developing positive attitudes towards postgraduate education.

VT curriculum

Rodgers has summarised the curriculum to be:

• the sum of teaching methods and content
• a body of knowledge to which the learner must be exposed
• the sum of all planned activities and experiences to which the learner may be exposed to achieve learning goals (Rodgers, 1986).

The ideal curriculum should:

• be learner-centred
• enthuse and empower the learner rather than merely inform
• explore concepts and values as well as facts
• contain a statement of aims for each session
• be as interactive as possible
• use multiple, and a variety of, methods to deliver the content.

With this in mind, Guilbert's (1997) four Cs model of curriculum development is both relevant and practical to the design of the study course:

• Co-operation – the curriculum requires the input of VDPs, advisers, trainers and all those involved in the process

- Continuous – the curriculum needs to evolve continuously
- Comprehensive – the curriculum needs to be a tool that helps direct learners when devising their learning goals
- Concrete – the curriculum needs to be specific with a well-defined set of objectives.

In undergraduate teaching, the curriculum reflects the published syllabus for a particular part of the course and students undertake examinations at the end of the period of teaching. This traditional approach is teacher-centred.

In contrast, because vocational training is learner-centred, it has been suggested that the content of the curriculum should include three elements (Samuel, 1990):

1 facts
2 concepts
3 values.

Facts can be learned from books so the purpose of the VT study days must be to present factual information in:

- the context of previous experience, and
- a way that can be applied to new situations and circumstances.

Facts will now convert to *knowledge* and the purpose of the curriculum is to facilitate this process. To paraphrase a popular anecdote, education is what is left when the taught facts have been forgotten.

The *concepts* that support vocational training include:

- responsibility for self-development on the part of the VDP
- commitment to life-long learning
- an understanding of underlying methodology, e.g. experiential learning, learning styles
- respect for the patient's autonomy.

The VT curriculum should also help VDPs to develop and explore their own *values* and how they relate to the values and beliefs held by others. This is an important aspect of the taught course. The exploration and definition of values emerges from the principles of experiential learning.

Another useful model of the curriculum is the Skilbeck model, which includes five components:

1 situation analysis

2 goal formulation: general and specific objectives
3 programme building
4 interpretation and implementation
5 evaluation.

(Skilbeck, 1975)

This model recognises all the different facets of vocational training and encompasses all the key principles.

The VT adviser is responsible for the content of the curriculum, but there is general agreement that the content should fall within the guidance published by CVT. Many trainers and VDPs play an active role in curriculum development in vocational training. Feedback at trainers' meetings and in-practice evidence will undoubtedly assist the VT adviser in curriculum planning.

The regional adviser and/or the postgraduate dental dean are required to review and approve the programme content prior to its official publication. A copy is sent to all trainers and VDPs. CVT also receives a copy of the programme from all schemes and has a task group that surveys a selection to ensure that it broadly reflects CVT's curriculum guidance.

Time is usually set aside for group work during which trainees are able to share experiences and discuss items of topical interest. The VT adviser normally oversees the group work.

An indication of the broad range of subjects covered in the course is given in Table 11.1. This is not an exhaustive list but it gives a broad view

Table 11.1 Typical content of the study course

Term 1 *General overview*	Term 2 *Improving quality of care*	Term 3 *New horizons*
Administration • structure of NHS • forms • regulations • medico-legal aspects of dental practice • basic practice management • personal finance	**Administration** • basics of financial management • time management • self-management • visits to DPB, GDC, BDA • communication skills • dealing with difficult patients	**Administration** • legal aspects of general dental practice • staff employment and motivation • stress management • practice management systems • finance and investment • business skills
Clinical • history, diagnosis and treatment planning • psychology of dental care • management of emergencies • evidence-based dentistry • clinical governance	**Clinical** • advancing clinical skills • revision of core skills including hands-on training • new techniques and methods • critical appraisal of new methods and materials	**Clinical** • new ideas and concepts • advance treatment planning **Continuing professional education** • career choices and options • postgraduate education

of the subjects that would be covered. No two VT courses are alike and the content, particularly of the second and third terms, can vary from scheme to scheme and from year to year, depending on the needs and wants of the VDPs. It is not possible to cover all subjects in equal depth given the fixed duration of the study course.

The early part of the course focuses on the organisation of the National Health Service with particular reference to the GDS, treatment planning, radiography, emergency procedures, basic practice administration and guidance on problem solving and handling difficult situations.

Relationships between the dentist and his or her dental team and patients are explored in sessions covering communication skills. In the second term, the emphasis shifts towards hands-on clinical dentistry with an emphasis on advancing the clinical skills taught at undergraduate level.

The third term explores horizons new to most trainees. The complex fields of accountancy, insurance, finance and advanced business and practice management are just some examples of the subjects covered.

The limited time available for the study days means that there will be some subjects that cannot be covered in any great depth. VDPs are encouraged to pursue their interests through further personal investigation with the help of their trainers. Clinical photography is just one example where it is impossible to give anything more than an overview of the subject in the time available.

In addition to this teaching, scheme organisers may also arrange visits to other practices, dental laboratories and various professional organisations. These visits are designed to broaden the trainee's perspectives, and to give them an understanding of how key organisations and professional bodies interrelate and support the general dental practitioner.

Evaluation

Evaluation has been defined as 'a formal or disciplined approach to examine the value of a program based not only on its outcomes but also on its context, inputs, processes and procedures and products' (Worthen and Sanders, 1987). This is sometimes referred to as the CIPP model. It is a process of inquiry that includes the development of criteria and standards for evaluation as well as the collection of relevant data; a comparison of the two will then help to determine quality and is conducted for the purposes of quality assurance.

The difference between evaluation and assessment is that the participant or the organisation generates the value response to an evaluation procedure, while assessment relies on the trainer or tutor setting the value system.

Study course evaluation is important for a number of reasons. Its aim is:

- to involve and motivate VDPs
- to provide feedback to the presenter for his or her own satisfaction
- to assist in curriculum development
- to gather suggestions and ideas that may prove useful in later sessions
- to communicate with others in the organisation
- to exchange opinions and ideas with other courses.

Kirkpatrick (1959) identifies four types of evaluation. These are:

1 reaction
2 learning
3 behaviour (performance)
4 results (impact).

Trainers have a key role to play in the information gathering process relating to (3) and occasionally (4) but may also be involved in (1) and (2) if they are presenting on the course.

Box 11.1 Evaluation

Please take a few minutes to complete this evaluation questionnaire. Your comments provide the organisers with useful feedback, which plays an important part in the planning of future courses. Thank you for your co-operation.

Date: **Title of presentation:**   **Presented by:**

What aspects of this study day have been most useful to you?

What have you learned today?

How will today change the way you practise?

Please make other comments in the space below.

Reaction evaluation

This requires feedback from the VDPs immediately after the session. This information is obtained by using an 'evaluation form', which asks certain questions of the learner.

There is usually a rating scale of 1–5, which produces a numerical result, which can be aggregated and makes for easy comparisons. An alternative is to use a questionnaire that does not use numerical ratings but asks the learner to indicate which words best describe their reaction to the presentation.

Learning evaluation

The learning evaluation is designed to discover what principles, techniques and facts have been understood and absorbed by the VDP. The learning evaluation is not concerned with how those principles, techniques and facts will be translated into the practising environment. By asking different and more specific questions, a learning evaluation is carried out and the responses are more objective. Box 11.1 gives one simple, but surprisingly effective, example of the open question format.

Other questions that might be asked are:

- *How much of the information presented was new to you?*
- *Identify three things that you have learned today.*
- *Give some examples of how today's presentation will influence the way you practise.*
- *In what ways do you now feel differently towards ...?*

Attitudes and values can be measured by making a number of statements and asking the learner to circle one of the following in relation to each statement. The statements invite the learner to rate the course in the following way:

1 = strongly disagree
2 = disagree
3 = neither agree nor disagree
4 = agree
5 = strongly agree.

Evaluation questionnaires can be subdivided into sections to include questions on:

- content
- design

- the presenter
- environment
- results.

Examples of questions from each section include:

- I was well informed about the objectives of this course
- the course was relevant to general dental practice
- the presenter was well prepared
- the training facility was comfortable
- I will be able to use the information I learned in everyday practice.

A similar design of questionnaire can also be used in reaction evaluation.

Performance evaluation
The impact of a study session on the VDP's practical performance can only be measured at practice level and trainers are ideally placed to review this. Performance evaluation feedback is important to VT advisers and there will be opportunities during the year for trainers to feed back their views on VDP performance. In practice, it is very difficult to measure. Kirkpatrick offered some guidelines for evaluating training in terms of behavioural changes (Kirkpatrick, 1959). These were:

- conduct a systematic appraisal of on-the-job performance on a before-and-after basis
- the appraisal of performance should be made by one or more of the following groups (the more the better): trainees, supervisors, subordinates and others familiar with the trainee's on-the-job performance
- conduct a statistical analysis to compare before-and-after performance to relate changes to training
- conduct post-training appraisal three months or more after training so that trainees have an opportunity to put into practice what they have learned. Subsequent appraisals may add to the validity of the study.

This list can be adapted to general practice and experienced trainers will recognise the impact of this approach in the design and recommended use of the professional development portfolio. The reference to 'trainees' in this list is intended as a generic description.

Impact evaluation
This is perhaps the most valuable evaluation method, but the most difficult to implement within VT. It is designed to measure the long-term effectiveness of the training programme by identifying which elements of

vocational training have a significant and lasting impact on the future practising habits of VDPs. This information would be most useful for the future development of vocational training because it would help to answer the following important questions:

- How effective is vocational training in education terms?
- Is it cost-effective?
- How can it be improved?

The evidence regarding the long-term impact of vocational training is not conclusive.

Multi-source evaluation

Multi-source evaluation is an example of 360-degree feedback, which has been defined as 'the systematic collection and feedback of performance data on an individual or group, derived from a number of stakeholders in their performance' (Ward, 1997). It permits the gathering of information from numerous sources, all of whom may be regarded as stakeholders in vocational training. They include VDPs, speakers, trainers, VT advisers, course administrators and, of course, patients. The process is a tool to facilitate the development of VT at a local and national level. Trainers will be asked for their opinions and comments on aspects of vocational training at various stages of the training year. Some may sit as representatives on national committees and task groups and participate in the process of 360-degree feedback.

The purpose of 360-degree feedback is:

- to align individual and group expectations with the aims and objectives of VT
- to support a commitment to continuous learning
- to provide reliable and useful performance measures
- to encourage an evidence-based approach to training
- to review current methodology.

There are a number of ways in which this could be achieved. These include:

1 *Anecdotal information* – There is a temptation to try and quantify value and assign a numerical score to a process even though there are inherent flaws in this approach. It should be remembered that subjective evidence could be equally valuable when used in combination with other measures.

2 *Peer review* – The peer review process manifests itself in the form of the quality assessment framework, which is used by CVT in its visits to regions.

3 *Focus groups* – From time to time focus groups are convened to look at a particular aspect of vocational training. For example, CVT has a focus group, which studies the design, structure and content of the study days by reviewing the course programmes from schemes throughout the country. It reports back with ideas and suggestions and disseminates examples of good practice.

4 *Questionnaires* – The use of questionnaires has already been discussed in an earlier section.

5 *Formative review* – The professional development portfolio is an important tool for formative review.

6 *Records and files* – A review of records and other documentation can give useful information on administrative processes in place and their effectiveness. This method, amongst others, is used by CVT in their quality assurance programme.

Does VT work?

The purpose of evaluating the course is, in many ways, an attempt at answering this perplexing question. The question was posed by Pereira Gray in his review of vocational training in medical practice and the conclusion was that there was no available evidence that vocationally trained practitioners provided a better standard of care than those who did not undertake VT (Pereira Gray, 1979). This poses what is essentially a measurement dilemma – a dilemma identified by Albert Einstein who famously commented that 'not everything that counts can be counted and not everything that can be counted counts'.

A controlled study would be the only way to find out and clearly this is not a practical solution given the numerous personality factors, which could not be matched in comparing the performance of groups of individuals. Given the inherent difficulties in adopting this approach, existing methodology aims to answer some key questions. These are:

- *What happens during the training year – in the tutorial and on the study days?*
  Observation techniques can be used to record activities and interactions.
- *What goals have been set for the year and are they achieved?*
  Goal setting is an important feature of the VT year. Behavioural change is triggered by the goal setting which arises from feedback and not the feedback itself.

- *How can teaching be improved?*
  CVT undertakes a quality assurance programme of all the regions in the country to ensure that standards are maintained.

Some of these issues are likely to be addressed in CVT's forthcoming review of vocational training, which commenced in July 2001.

Training and learning must be seen to have value. It is not enough to review experiences but it is more useful to see what behavioural changes have taken place as a result of the training programme. In one review of why VDPs enjoy a training event (Rattan, 1998), it was noted that VDPs found particular sessions inspiring and beneficial but this did not necessarily lead to changes at practice level.

In a recent paper, Ralph *et al.* (2001) noted that 74% of VDP respondents said that VT had encouraged them to continue with their professional development (CPD) against 54% of non-VDP respondents, but the other CPD activities of the two groups were very similar.

The broader aspects of VT need to be constantly reviewed in the light of these observations.

CHAPTER 12

Trainers' meetings

Trainer meetings are important events in the vocational training calendar. They are arranged by the VT adviser to monitor and review progress during the training year and are normally held at least once each term at the postgraduate centre. The purpose of trainer meetings is to:

- provide a supportive framework for trainers
- exchange ideas and opinions
- discuss problems and solutions
- help plan future course content
- receive feedback on VDP progress and curriculum content
- discuss matters of general interest.

One of the great strengths of the vocational training scheme is the peer group support enjoyed by VDPs and trainers alike. It is the trust and mutual respect that bonds the group and creates the synergy and camaraderie enjoyed by so many trainers. Trainers are encouraged to maintain this relationship throughout the year and to use the trainer meeting as the focal event for sharing experiences.

In some regions, the trainer group may elect or nominate a group representative through whom important communications can be channelled outside the meetings and who may also act as a co-ordinator of any social events that may take place.

Trainers can play a major role in curriculum development for the study days. Advisers will seek feedback from trainers to see to what extent the study days are influencing the VDP's in-practice behaviour. The role of the trainer in this process is shown in Figure 12.1.

Meeting agenda

An agenda for discussion will be circulated to all trainers prior to the meeting. Group leaders may wish to use the agenda listing as a tool to curtail unwanted discussion. All matters arising remain confidential to

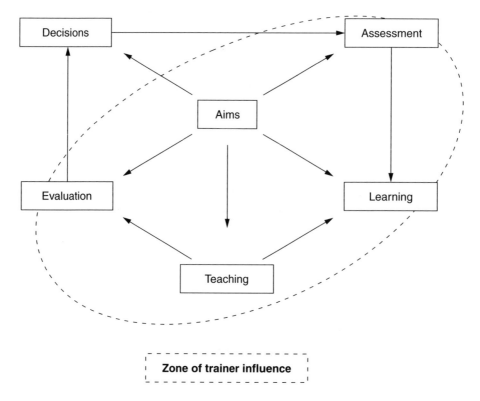

Figure 12.1 The trainer's potential zone of influence in curriculum development (adapted from Cowan and Harding, 1986).

group members, unless there is unanimous agreement to circulate information or observations to a wider audience. If individual members wish to raise certain matters in private with the VT adviser, they are at liberty to do so and confidentiality is assured.

Trainer workshops

In addition to local scheme-related meetings, many regions organise a variety of workshops on all aspects of vocational training and related subjects. New trainers will be expected to attend induction courses designed to familiarise them with all aspects of VT; experienced trainers can also attend courses. The number of days allocated for these activities varies from region to region, but will normally be no more than three or four. First-time trainers are normally required to attend more days as part of their induction programme.

Induction training is for general dental practitioners who have little or no experience in vocational training. The content is aimed at giving trainers an insight into their role and responsibilities, and to expand on all aspects of vocational training. Experienced trainers may be invited to participate, or to act as facilitators on these days. These courses are normally held at the beginning of the training year and before the start of the trainee's scheme study days. All newly appointed trainers are expected to attend.

A number of courses are also organised for experienced trainers. They cover a wide range of subject matter ranging from health and safety updates to courses on teaching techniques and methods.

Confidentiality

The content of discussions at trainer meetings can be wide-ranging and frequently involves an in-depth analysis of VDP performance. There will be sensitive clinical issues to be discussed, financial information to be shared and some anecdotal quips just for good measure. It is esssential that trainers respect the strict confidentiality of this forum for discussion so that the discussions that take place are confined to those who are present and not relayed back to individual VDPs.

CHAPTER 13

Communication skills

Many of the difficulties and problems that arise between the trainer and the VDP are the result of a breakdown in communication. In fact, many complaints against dentists result for the same reason. Many of these difficulties are avoidable if people have a better understanding of the process of communication and how it relates to the psychology of human behaviour.

The communication process

The essential components of the communication process are shown in Figure 13.1. The Shannon-Weaver model of communication is a typical example of a so-called transmission model of communication. Principally concerned with communication technology, and first proposed in 1949, it is a widely used model for the study of human communication. It identifies the six key elements of the communication process. One of the limitations of the model was its linearity because it saw communication as a one-way process. The introduction of the feedback loop, which can have a direct bearing on how the source presents further information, overcomes the limitation of the original concept.

An understanding of the process will help trainers to avoid many problems associated with communication breakdown, and facilitate the teaching of good communication skills to their VDPs.

Anything that obstructs information transmission is a barrier to effective communication. The removal of these barriers improves the quality of communication. The most common barriers to good communication are:

• message distortion
• information overload
• semantic misinterpretation
• noise.

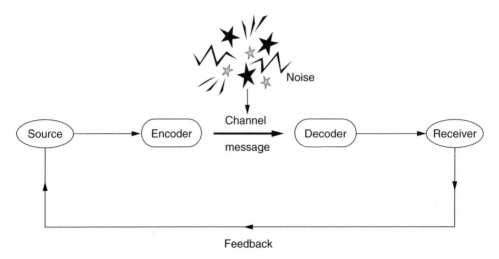

Figure 13.1   The Shannon-Weaver model of communication.

Message distortion

Message distortion can occur where there is no direct communication between the source and receiver. The message is relayed via an interme-diate source or sources, which can result in the final message being rather different than intended by the original source.

In a busy practice, chains of communication are essential for efficient practice management. Indeed, the whole concept of a team management relies on good communication amongst the members of the dental team.

Nevertheless, misunderstandings can sometimes arise and lead to interpersonal conflict. To avoid this happening between the trainer and the VDP, direct communication between these parties is advised, partic-ularly when sensitive issues are involved. It is very tempting for a trainer to pass a casual but critical remark to a nurse or receptionist only to discover later that the message has been relayed to the VDP, but in a distorted way.

Direct communication will prevent misunderstandings arising from message distortion.

Information overload

Too much information delivered too quickly causes overload. Important information may therefore be overlooked, or simply not received.

Trainers should aim to avoid information overload at all times. There is always a temptation to cover as many aspects of practice organisation as quickly as possible or to discuss complex issues hastily in between patients. In these circumstances, the risk of overload is high and a lot of what is being said is simply lost in thin air.

To avoid this, complex communications should be delivered at a pace that gives the trainee time to absorb what is being said.

Semantic misinterpretation

The use of imprecise or incorrect phraseology can result in incomprehensible messages. The use of technical words and jargon is not always appropriate when communicating with patients.

Experienced practitioners are well aware of this problem, but trainees may require guidance in how to communicate effectively with their patients. For example, many find it difficult to discuss treatment costs, or have difficulty in explaining the treatment plan in a way that facilitates the patient's understanding and acceptance of it.

These skills can be learned. The trainer may invite his or her trainee to sit in during a clinical session and observe how these difficulties are surmounted.

Noise

In this context, 'noise' is a term used to describe any distracting influences, which hinder the receipt of the message. For example, repeated interruptions during a tutorial will distract both parties, and compromise the quality of communication. The interruptions constitute 'noise'.

Avoid noise by conducting important communications, such as tutorials, in protected time and away from distractions.

Models of interaction

There are many 'models' of human interaction and they are characterised by different approaches to the subject. It is beyond the scope of this text to review these in any depth, but there are two that are particularly relevant to vocational training given the relationship between the trainer and the VDP. These are:

* transactional analysis
* neuro-linguistic programming.

Transactional analysis (TA)

Transactional analysis gained nationwide popularity in the 1960s as a result of Eric Berne's book *Games People Play* (Berne, 1969). Its popularity grew during the 1970s and more books were written on the subject. Today, the concept is regarded by some as outdated but there is a core of information, which trainers will find useful in their relationships with the VDPs. Many believe that Eric Berne's book, *What Do You Say After You Say Hello,* should be essential reading for all those whose profession relies on human interaction (Berne, 1975).

Many have found TA a useful tool in understanding the complexities of professional and personal relationships. A transaction is defined as a unit of interaction between people, which comprises a stimulus and a response. The units of interaction are rarely discrete but form part of a set. Some of these sets can be productive and healthy, but others can be destructive and unhealthy; transactional analysis is a psychological theory about the feelings of people, their thinking and their behaviour. The concept is shrouded in jargon, but it should not deter the reader from understanding the brief explanations given in this text.

The basic theory professes that when people interact they do so in one of three different ego-states. These are:

- parent ego-state
- child ego-state
- adult ego-state.

These states represent patterns of behaviour and are present to a greater or lesser extent in all individuals. People can behave from their parent ego-state or the child ego-state or the adult ego-state. Different ego-states will tend to dominate in different situations.

Experienced trainers will immediately recognise one or other of these from previous trainer–trainee relationships. An understanding of this concept will lead to an ability to recognise the different states and the circumstances in which one or other tends to dominate will help trainers to better relate to and understand the nature of the trainer–VDP relationship.

The parent ego-state
The parent in us derives from memories of what children see in their parents or equivalent authority figures. These figures are providers of 'how to' information, of regulations and rules (the 'dos and don'ts' of our environment). The vocabulary used in parent-type communication will be rich in terms such as 'should', 'never', 'always', etc. The parent judges

for or against and can be controlling or supportive. If the parent is seen as critical, it is called the 'critical parent' and when it is supportive it is called the 'nurturing parent'. The comparisons are very pertinent to the trainer–VDP relationship.

The child ego-state

When people are in the child ego-state they tend to act like the child they once were. The child can be observed in children for prolonged periods of time, but can also be seen in adults in certain situations where people have 'permission to let the child out', such as at sports events and parties. It is worth noting that the child will also appear for prolonged periods of time in the form of depression or grief.

The adult ego-state

This is the rational, objective and logical face of human behaviour. It focuses on analytical thought, reasoned argument, and information processing and decision making, and relies on the separation of an individual from his or her emotions. A very important part of the adult ego-state is to predict outcomes and to provide fact-based solutions to situations that may develop around the person. It should be noted that this fact-based critical approach is fundamentally different from the approach adopted in the critical parent state, which is value-based.

Type of transactions

When people relate to each other, a transaction is said to have taken place. Trainers and VDPs will encounter each other in a variety of situations and circumstances during the training year. There are a number of transaction types:

Complimentary transactions involve one ego-state in each person. In a crossed transaction, the response is addressed to an ego-state that is different from the one that started the stimulus. Crossed transactions disrupt communication and analysts often remark that 'whenever a disruption of communication occurs, a crossed transaction caused it'.

Covert transactions are said to occur when people say one thing and mean another and are intentionally deceptive. TA encourages people to be honest with themselves and with each other about their feelings, rather than covert.

Transactional analysis theory observes that people take up one or other of four life positions:

- Position 1: I'm not OK – You're OK.

- Position 2: I'm not OK – You're not OK.
- Position 3: I'm OK – You're not OK.
- Position 4: I'm OK – You're OK.

These life positions reflect the stances people adopt in their transactions, and experienced trainers will recognise many of them. The relationship between trainer and VDP depends on the life position adopted.

Transactional analysis theory suggests that in childhood the dominant position is position 1. At about the age of three years, this position is either confirmed, or there may be a shift to position 2 or 3. This new position then remains fixed, unless the individual makes a conscious effort to change to position 4, the adult to adult ego-state.

Trainers should be aware of the life positions assumed by their VDPs. The position will be a direct reflection on their attitude towards their work and to dental practice in general. Some observations concerning these positions are as follows.

- *Position 1: I'm not OK – You're OK.* This is the role of the 'loser' who sees all events around him or her as failures and is unable to recognise success. He or she always sees everyone else as OK, thereby accentuating their own perception of self-failure even more.
- *Position 2: I'm not OK – You're not OK.* This is characterised by feelings of unworthiness and of not being wanted. This person will be withdrawn, have a tendency to drop out and put in the minimum effort to get by in life.
- *Position 3: I'm OK – You're not OK.* This individual has the characteristics of a tough taskmaster. Others are always blamed for set backs. Self-blame never enters the equation.
- *Position 4: I'm OK – You're OK.* This position is unique because it is a position that the individual consciously tries to adopt, unlike the other three. It encourages feelings of self-respect and respect for others. The individual favours a co-operative and teamwork approach to management.

Position 4 relies on conscious effort and forms the basis of good trainer–trainee relationships.

Table 13.1 summarises the characteristics of life positions and how they relate to behaviour at work. Many of the aspects discussed in this table apply equally to the trainer's and the VDP's own life positions.

A VDP with a negative life position, such as life position 1, may struggle for success during the training year. By providing the VDP with an understanding of transactional analysis theory, behaviour can be influenced, and it should encourage a conscious shift towards life position 4.

Table 13.1 How life position influences behaviour at work (based on Berne, 1969)

	Feels towards others	Communi-cates	Responds to delegation	Develops	Handles disagree-ment	Deals with problems	Spends time	Acts
1 **I'm not OK – You're OK**	Inferior	Defensively, self-depre-cating	Fearfully	Slowly – needs reassurance and help	Sees the prob-lem as due to his own inad-equacy	By relying on others	Either brood-ing or in over-activity	By the book; is afraid to use initiative
2 **I'm not OK – You're not OK**	Alienated, despondent	With hostility and abruptness	By trying to avoid dele-gated tasks; accepts responsibility reluctantly	With difficulty; withdraws and repeatedly makes mistakes	By either avoid-ing or worsen-ing the conflict; by involving other people	By giving in	Withdrawing, playing 'games'	Does the minimum he can get away with
3 **I'm OK – You're not OK**	Superior	Defensive but aggressive	By delaying tactics and argument	With difficulty; unwilling to learn from others	By blaming others	By rejecting others' ideas	Boasting, provoking others	When forced; may ask for official instructions
4 **I'm OK – You're OK**	Equal	Openly	Readily	Independently; learns willingly	By facing the issue and solving the problem mutually	By consulta-tion or by trusting own judgement	Productively taking action when neces-sary	On own ini-tiative when not given work

Neuro-linguistic programming (NLP)

NLP has been defined as 'the study of human excellence', or 'the study of subjective experience'. The word *neuro* relates to the five senses through which individuals perceive the world around them and linguistic refers to language, including non-verbal cues, through which neural representations are coded and given meaning.

NLP is useful in communication, management of change, mental management and personal/professional development. It is a constantly evolving set of models, presuppositions, patterns, techniques and observation-based theories resulting from observation, the structure of subjective experiences, behaviour and communication.

A presupposition is an assumption of truth on which individuals will act. Some of the fundamental presuppositions of NLP that may impact on the way trainers interact with the VDP are listed below.

- *The map is not the territory* – This phrase was coined by Alfred Korzybski, a well-respected scholar of semantics, whose work provided the tools to improve our evaluation of 'reality'. The principle is best illustrated by considering someone who travels to work by car and who regularly uses a mental map to get there. The choice of route is always the same and conforms to the mental map of the journey. As this process continues month after month and year after year, the mental map remains the same but new road systems may have sprung up in the meantime. Unless the driver makes a conscious effort to update the mental map, he or she will continue in the same old way. Others, who have updated their mental map, may have found useful short cuts or less stressful routes. The same principle can be applied to the way professionals perceive their profession – change the map and the reality changes at the same time.
- *Behind every behaviour is a positive intention* – All behavioural responses have a positive aspect to them, including those that may seem irrational – someone shouting in order to be heard or someone deploying avoidance tactics to feel safe are just two examples. NLP seeks to distil the positive intent from the situation.
- *There is no such thing as failure, there is only feedback* – Every response is useful. It may not be what you wanted to hear, but the knowledge gained from it is invaluable.
- *In any system, the element with the most flexibility exerts the most influence* – Put simply, this statement is saying that choice is better than no choice.
- *If one person can do something, then anyone can learn it* – This presupposition puts forward the view that the skills of decision making, creativity

and confidence can all be learned and reminds us that there is a structure to achievement, which can be learned.

- *People already have all the resources they need* – This suggests that the resources for achievement are already there and have to be accessed.
- *If what you are doing isn't working, then do something different* – There is a tendency for people to 'do more of the same' when things do not go according to plan or are not working out. The tendency is to try harder with the same approach, but NLP tells us to do something different and try a different approach. The limitations are in the mental map and not the territory.
- *The meaning of communication is the response you get* – Others (the receivers) interpret the communication in relation to their mental map and not the mental map of the sender. If the sender notices how the communication is received, then he or she can modify the message to ensure that what is meant is said and what is received is meant and said!

NLP uses the word 'rapport' to describe a relationship of trust and responsiveness. Individuals vary in the experiences and perceptions of the world and exhibit different values and beliefs. In order to establish rapport people need to 'get inside' the world of others and acknowledge their view. This does not mean that you have to agree with it, just that it must be recognised and respected. Rapport is established in face-to-face interactions through words, voice tone and body language. The impact of body language and voice tone has been shown to have a major impact on the perception of trustworthiness by others. If there is an obvious conflict between the words that are spoken and the body language that accompanies them, the receiver will pay more attention to the non-verbal element of the communication.

Practitioners of NLP say that it facilitates:

- self-discovery
- finding hidden resources within oneself
- the change of unwanted behaviour
- achievement
- handling events that were formerly frustrating
- creation of rapport with peers, patients and family.

Experience suggests that many trainers use some or many of the principles discussed here in VT, but may not necessarily be aware that they reflect the presuppositions of NLP. It is a model that has been recommended when planning the VDP's learning needs (Chambers and Wall, 2000). It should be noted that some authorities challenge aspects of NLP and question its reliability and validity. For example, Robert Todd Carol of the Skeptics Dictionary website (http://skeptic.com) states that 'NLP makes claims about thinking and perception which do not seem to be supported by neuroscience'. He goes on to state that 'this is not to say that the techniques don't work ... they may work and work quite well, but there is no way of knowing whether the claims behind their origin are valid'. The reader is referred to the numerous specialist texts on the subject for a more in-depth discussion.

CHAPTER 14

Financial aspects of VT

The financial implications of vocational training can be divided into three categories, which are:

- arrangements for VDPs
- arrangements for trainers
- practice income and expenditure in relation to VT.

Arrangements for VDPs

The arrangements for VDPs can be summarised as follows.

- They are salaried employees of the practice and are paid in the same way as all other employees. The pay scale is fixed, and the trainer normally receives notification of any changes to remuneration.
- It is a legal requirement to provide VDPs with an itemised payslip to show gross pay, National Insurance, superannuation deductions (unless he or she chooses to opt out of the scheme), any variable deductions and the net pay. National Insurance deductions differ from those of other staff and are on a contracted-out basis for the VDP. Tax tables can be obtained from the local tax office.
- PAYE and National Insurance are deducted and trainers are required to open a tax deduction form as they would for any employee.
- Many VDPs will not have a P45. In this situation, the Inland Revenue requires the employer to complete a P46 form. These are sent together (or separately if the employee wishes) to the tax office who will issue a P45 with the correct tax code. It is advisable to do this as soon as a VDP has been appointed to expedite the notification of their tax code.
- The trainer pays the VDP's salary. The trainer is reimbursed at a later date.

Arrangements for trainers

The financial arrangements for trainers can be summarised as follows.

- Trainers receive a monthly training grant, which is paid one month in arrears from the Dental Practice Board. The training grant is equivalent to 15% of what was formerly TANI (target average net income) for dentists. This is paid on the trainer's monthly schedule from the Dental Practice Board.
- All fees (NHS and private income) resulting from the VDP's clinical work accrue to the practice.
- The VDP's salary, together with the employer's National Insurance contribution, is reimbursed to the trainer by the Dental Practice Board and appears as an additional item on the DPB schedule. It is reimbursed one month in arrears. It should be noted that the DPB can only pay this after they have received the necessary authorisation from the Health Authority. The Health Authority will issue form FP81 on receipt of the Confirmation of Approval as Trainer Certificate, which is sent to trainers by the deanery once they have been appointed. Form FP81 should be completed and returned to the Health Authority who will then advise the Dental Practice Board to put in place the arrangements for reimbursement and the grant. Any delay in completion of this essential paperwork will inevitably result in delayed reimbursement.
- Expenses incurred for attending study days and trainer meetings and other VT related activities are reclaimable from the local Health Authority on submission of form FP84.

Box 14.1 shows the key facts that are circulated to all trainers when the salary and grant structure changes.

Practice income/expenditure in relation to VT

Dental practices are small businesses and must contend with the commercial pressures common to all other small businesses. The placement of a VDP into this environment is a test not only of teaching skills, but also of the business skills essential to run and manage a successful practice.

There is a baseline cost attached to running the VDP's surgery and these must be met. There are no guarantees that this will happen and it is therefore important that performance measures reflect the financial aspects of vocational training. It would be inappropriate for trainers to

Box 14.1   Key facts on finance

IMPORTANT NOTICE

VOCATIONAL TRAINING FOR GENERAL DENTAL PRACTICE

FACTS ON FINANCE

The following increases to salaries and grants has occurred:

TRAINEE SALARY is **£2,009.00** per month from April 1, 2001
TRAINER GRANT is **£601.00** per month from April 1, 2001

Amendment number 85 to the Statement of Dental Remuneration, recently circulated to dentists, authorised the payment of the above increases **as from April 1, 2001**.

TRAINEE'S SALARY

Trainee's gross pay	Superannuation deduction	Net pay for income tax	National Insurance Employee's Contribution Contracted-out Table D (based on gross pay)
£2,009.00	£120.54	£1888.46	£137.09

TRAINER'S CLAIM TO DPB

	£0.00
Trainer's grant	£601.00
Trainee's salary	£2,009.00
Employer's NI contribution	£145.25
TOTAL	**£2,755.25**

DPB RE-IMBURSEMENT TO TRAINER

	£0.00
Above amount	£2,755.25
Less employee's Superannuation contribution	£120.54
TOTAL RE-IMBURSED	**£2634.71**

N.B.

The amount deducted for the trainer's Superannuation contribution in respect of the trainer's grant varies according to the total fees earned.

The NI contributions quoted above are at contracted-out rates from Table D. The code number for "Contracted-out Health Service Workers" (ECON) is **E3900000M**, and the NHS Scheme Contracted-out number (SCON) is **S2730000B**.

CVT Office, 123 Gray's Inn Road, London, WC1X 8WD
Telephone: 020 7905 1207 Facsimile: 020 7905 1212
Email: shall@eastman.ucl.ac.uk URL: http://www.eastman.ucl.ac.uk/cvt/

focus solely on this aspect of performance, and particularly so in the early stages of training, but VDPs do need to be made aware of the financial aspects of general dental practice as the year progresses.

It is the experience of many trainers that the VT year can be divided into four quarters for the purposes of financial planning. In quarter 1, there is every likelihood that the VDP will be working at a loss. Within quarters 2 and 3 there will be a gradual and sustained shift towards profitability and the fourth quarter tends to compensate for the earlier months.

A typical, but schematic, financial profile is shown in Figure 14.1. Schedules will continue to arrive under the VT contract number for at least three months beyond the date of expiry of the contract. This is reflected in the steep decline in revenue shown by the dotted line.

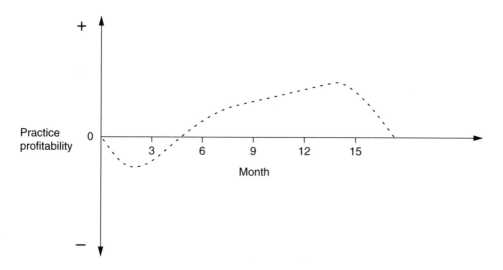

Figure 14.1   Typical pattern of profit/loss during the VT year.

Comparisons

Trainers frequently use fee income data to compare VDP performance with that of their peers on the scheme for the current year or with the previous VDPs in preceding years. Comparisons are meaningful only if they are on a like-for-like basis.

Some VDPs begin their VT year with a pre-existing patient list from either a previous VDP or an outgoing associate. The continuing care and capitation payments will be payable on the VDP's contract number from the date of transfer and can skew any performance data based on gross fee income.

If the gross fee income from a VDP who has a patient list from the outset is compared with someone who has no list there will be a significant difference between their scheduled gross fee incomes. The variations can be quite dramatic, as illustrated in the two graphs in Figures 14.2 and 14.3, which summarise data from two VDPs. Their practising profiles were remarkably similar for the item of service work, but their performance, at a first glance, seemed to vary quite markedly (Figure 14.2). The difference could be accounted for in continuing care and capitation payments. With these payments excluded from the figures, the performances were in fact remarkably similar (Figure 14.3). The gross fee data relates to 1996 fee scales and is recorded after deduction of laboratory costs.

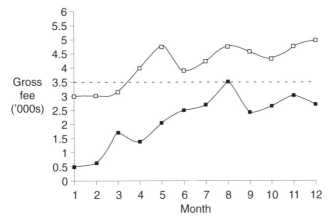

Figure 14.2 A comparison between two VDPs' gross NHS fee incomes less laboratory fees.

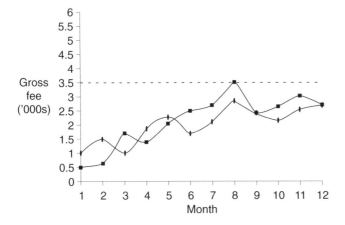

Figure 14.3 Gross fee income for the same two VDPs with capitation and continuing care fees excluded, i.e. item of service fees alone.

VDP involvement

New graduates entering general dental practice for the first time are largely unaware of the financial aspects of practice management, and will rely on their trainers to provide them with a better understanding of this complex subject. VDPs should have a working knowledge of the fundamental principles of financial management by the end of their training year. This is best achieved using any one of a number of structured and standardised formats.

In particular, VDPs ought to be familiar with three fundamental analyses as they apply to general dental practice:

* the break-even analysis
* analysis of expenditure
* schedule analysis.

Break-even analysis
A break-even graph is a useful tool for the analysis of practice costs and overheads as they relate to the practice fee income. The graph is compiled using basic information that all trainers should have or are able to get from a recent copy of the practice accounts.

VDPs will need to be familiar with the fundamental aspects of practice costs and revenue. The break-even analysis will help them to understand the basic concepts of fixed and variable costs as well as practice fee income.

* *The fixed costs* These will include mortgage or rent payments, lease payments, and practice development loans. The total figure is plotted on a graph and appears as a horizontal line F-F in Figure 14.4.
* *The variable costs* These relate to clinical activity within the practice. Examples include laboratory bills, dental materials costs and some staff costs. The variable costs are additional to fixed expenses and are entered on the graph as line FV. The sum of these two costs represents the total cost of running the practice.
* *The fee income* This is directly proportional to the work carried out. The relationship is between work done and fee income. This is shown as line OI.

The critical point on the graph is the intersection of line OI with line FV. This point of intersection, known as the break-even point, is shown as B on the graph, and is the point at which income exactly offsets expenditure. Anything above this line indicates profit and anything below it indicates a loss.

This is a useful exercise for discussing many aspects of practice finance

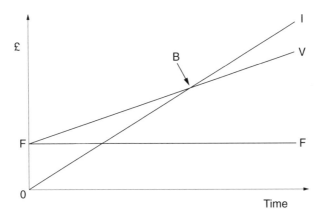

Figure 14.4   Break-even analysis.

with the VDP. Trainers may wish to set the VDPs the task of carrying out a break-even analysis of their own surgery, taking a proportion of total fixed costs for their calculations. Trainer assistance should be available for this exercise, which is a useful mechanism for learning about aspects of dental practice finance.

It is a good method of assessing how many of the basic principles the VDPs have understood.

Analysis of expenditure

An alternative way to discuss this subject is to analyse practice costs as a proportion of gross fee income. In this method, the absolute costs for a year are recorded. This information is easily obtainable from the practice accounts. The costs are then related to the gross fee income, and it is then possible to calculate the expenses of the practice per £1000 of fee income. Figure 14.5 shows the results of one such exercise that was carried out at a training practice in London. Interestingly, the ratio of expenses to profit was very close to the national average for that year.

Schedule analysis

VDPs should be familiar with schedule procedures. The key points to cover include:

- the overall schedule format
- the recording of item of service, continuing care and capitation payments
- list size information, including additions and deletions
- principles of schedule checking and how to avoid mistakes
- remission cases
- use of statistical information, e.g. cost per estimate

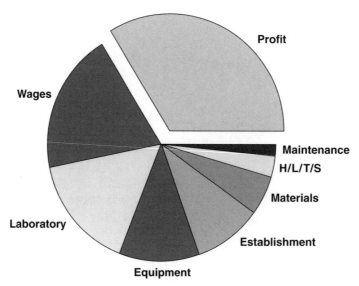

Figure 14.5 Earnings/expenses analysis.

- querying payments – procedures
- adjustments in patient charge
- deductions such as superannuation and LDC funds
- sample remuneration calculations as carried out for associates.

It is suggested that after an initial period of three months, VDPs should be given an opportunity of calculating their own fee income as they would if they were associates. This allows them to compare fee income with their current salary and is good training for the future when they will be responsible for checking their own payments and laboratory bills. A sample sheet is shown in Box 14.2.

It can be a confusing subject for many VDPs and it is recommended that the exercise be undertaken in stages, perhaps over three or four consecutive months, leaving the VDP to undertake his or her own checking procedures in, say, month 4, with the trainer's help if requested. The analysis should commence after the first few months of training has been completed. An early emphasis on financial management is inappropriate. After a few months, the schedule payments will be more consistent and the task becomes more meaningful.

The Dental Practice Board provides quarterly practising profiles for VDPs, but these are distributed only to those contracts with at least £1000 of activity because a profile based on a lesser amount is likely to be unrepresentative of true prescribing activity. An example is shown in Box 14.3. VDPs should be familiar with this document and the interpretation of the statistics contained therein.

Box 14.2   Sample spreadsheet for recording payments

	Jan-00	Feb-00	Mar-00	Apr-00	May-00	Jun-00	Jul-00	Aug-00	Sep-00	Oct-00	Nov-00	Dec-00
NHS gross fees												
Private gross fees												
BUPA/Denplan												
TOTAL GROSS FEES												
LABORATORY FEES												
*												
*												
*												
*												
TOTAL												
GROSS LESS LAB												
50%												
DEDUCTIONS												
Superannuation												
Stat. + Vol. levy												
Credit card 1.25%												
Debts												
Counter claim												
Charging errors												
Subsidy												
FINAL PAYMENT												
VT SALARY												

Box 14.3 Sample VDP quarterly prescribing profile
October 2000 to December 2000

QUARTERLY FINANCIAL DETAILS

Vocational trainees
earning at least £1000

	Your contract		Percentage breakdown		
			Quartiles		
			Lower	Upper	Average
	£	%	%	%	%
Capitation	320	5.80	0.90	12.22	10.02
Continuing care	147	2.66	1.46	6.87	5.96
Weighted entry	0	0.00	0.00	0.00	0.00
Item of service (adult)	4826	87.49	71.76	92.38	77.06
Item of service (child)	223	4.05	2.67	8.52	6.68
Transitional pj153 ayment	0	0.00	0.00	0.00	0.28
Total quarterly gross fees	**5517**	**100.0**			**100.00**

Patient registration at 31 December 2000		%	%	%	%
Capitation	85	33.73	19.89	34.17	29.08
Continuing care	167	66.27	65.83	80.11	70.92
Total	**252**	**100.00**			**100.00**

ADULT ITEM OF SERVICE

	Your contract	Vocational trainees earning at least £1000		
		Quartiles		
		Lower	Upper	Average
Average cost per claim £	27.74	31.12	63.09	39.08
Remission cases per hundred claims	5.78	15.23	40.43	25.82
Exempt cases per hundred claims	4.05	2.86	6.80	4.84
Total adult item of service claims	**173**	**46**	**195**	**133**

ADULT ITEM OF SERVICE TREATMENT INDICATORS

Rate per hundred adult item of service claims

	Your contract	Vocational trainees ~~earning at least £1000~~		
		Quartiles		
		Lower	Upper	Average
Diagnosis and/or prevention only	41.62	22.43	45.11	40.80
One of more small radiographs	43.93	29.25	60.60	37.00
Scaling & polish	65.90	26.31	52.97	44.75
Periodontal treatment: two or more visits	2.31	2.46	14.71	7.37
Claims with filling treatment	34.10	31.08	46.40	35.54
Teeth filled	50.87	51.33	105.41	67.47
Claims with root treatment	1.16	1.65	9.23	3.95
Teeth root filled	1.16	1.69	10.34	4.52
Teeth root filled per hundred teeth conserved	2.20	2.58	10.87	6.30
Claims with provision of crown(s)/inlays	1.16	1.20	6.57	3.34
Teeth crowned/with inlays	1.73	1.31	8.24	4.28
Claims involving extraction	2.31	4.80	13.39	8.08
Teeth extracted	2.31	5.88	20.81	11.99
Provision of synthetic resin dentures	0.00	1.82	7.21	3.93
Provision of bridges	0.58	0.00	0.52	0.37
Recalled attendance	0.00	0.00	0.00	0.12
Domiciliary visits	0.00	0.00	0.00	0.48

CHAPTER 15

Barriers to training

The barriers to VT can be considered under two separate headings. These are:

1 poor performance / under-achievement
2 stress-related issues.

Poor performance

SCOPME, in its second working paper on the educational aspects of performance, emphasised the need for all doctors and dentists to participate in a regular process of review. It identified a number of issues concerning performance (SCOPME, 1999).

- The whole area of reviewing professional performance is a difficult but not an impossible one.
- To make sound judgements about performance it is necessary to have shared and declared agreement about the standards to be achieved.
- Setting standards is difficult.
- Reviewing progress is sound from an educational point of view.
- When performance problems arise, colleagues need to feel empowered to take appropriate, supportive and constructive action and have the skills to do so.

The observations relate very closely to vocational training and the reader will recognise that many facets of each of these statements have been discussed in different sections of this book. The role of trainers is critical to successful management of the poorly performing VDP.

Poor performance is difficult to define because many of the assessment measures used are subjective. A trainer who has previously been a trainer to high achievers may have a baseline expectation far above that of somebody whose previous experiences have been less than ideal. Perceptions of performance vary from practice to practice, but in general terms poor performance may be tackled at four levels:

- personal
- professional
- organisational
- environmental.

Personal factors

These can be related to lack of motivation, poor self-image, attitude and belief structures.

Motivation theories
There are a number of theories of motivation, but the majority fall into one of two broad categories.

- *Content theories*, e.g. Maslow's hierarchy of needs and Herzberg's two-factor theory (Maslow, 1970; Herzberg, 1959).
- *Process theories*, e.g. equity theory, goal theory and expectancy theory.

Content theories focus on identifying needs. Process theories seek to explain actions and decipher why people behave in the way that they do in certain situations. The theories rely on an understanding of human needs and postulate that it is the satisfaction of these needs that determines much of human behaviour.

Content theories
1 *Maslow's hierarchy of needs*
The American psychologist AH Maslow (1908–1970) suggested that there were five drivers of human motivation. He proposed a hierarchy of needs and postulated that when a person has satisfied level 1 needs they step up to level 2 and when this group of needs is satisfied, they progress to the next step in the hierarchy. Figure 15.1 shows Maslow's concept of a hierarchical structure.

The main criticism of Maslow's theory is that there is little evidence to support it. The notion that all individuals strive for these categories has been challenged on the basis that there are cultural and other factors that determine needs and the Maslow model does not accommodate this. It has also been suggested that some individuals may seek to satisfy some higher level needs before all the lower level needs have been fulfilled.

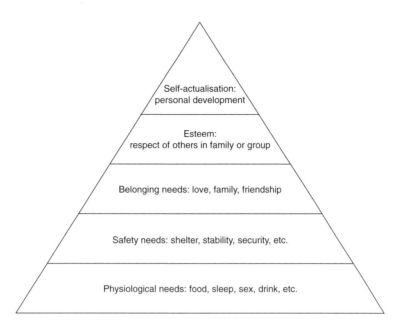

Figure 15.1 Maslow's hierarchy of needs.

2 *Herzberg's two-factor theory*

Herzberg has suggested that there are two sets of factors that determine human behaviour. One relates to the need to avoid pain/conflict and secure the basic necessities of life (equivalent to level 1 on Maslow's hierarchy) and the other focuses on personal development.

The theory was developed by questioning professional people to ascertain what most affected their behaviour and performance. Amongst the factors leading to dissatisfaction were:

- inadequate pay
- poor interpersonal relationships
- poor working conditions
- lack of fringe benefits.

These were known as 'hygiene factors'. (The medical analogy was based on the idea that hygiene promotes absence of disease but is not a cure in itself.) The hygiene factors in Herzberg's theory do not therefore increase job satisfaction, but they do at least prevent dissatisfaction. This has implications for general practice where poor relationships and work conditions can significantly demotivate members of the team.

In contrast, the motivating factors were those that improved job satisfaction and these included:

- sense of achievement
- recognition of effort from others in the organisation
- variety in work
- promotion prospects
- high levels of responsibility.

VDPs who have an active involvement in the organisation and management of the practice are likely to be better motivated and this will undoubtedly be reflected in their performance within the team.

The two-factor theory is noted for its proposal that pay is a hygiene factor rather than a motivating factor. This is an interesting observation given the fact that Herzberg's research focused on professional people at a managerial level.

Process theories
These are considered under the headings of:

- equity theory
- goal theory
- expectancy.

1 *Equity theory*
This deals with the feelings of employees and how they are treated compared with their colleagues in the workplace. If team members perceive that their reward-to-effort ratio is out of phase with others of perceived equal status within the practice, the result is unhappiness and discontentment. In this context, VDPs sometimes feel that they are poorly remunerated in comparison with other associates in the practice. Those affected by this perception will act in a way to reduce their cognitive dissonance.

The effects on the practice may include:

- absenteeism
- departure from employment
- disconcerted employees may act on others and cause behaviour changes in others.

The disconcerted VDP can influence other members of the peer group on the course and it has been the experience of some trainers that there have been particular instances when disenchantment has pervaded throughout the group for extended periods. The trainer meeting is an ideal medium to raise these sorts of issues.

When the rewards are perceived as equitable, motivation is restored.

2 *Goal theory*

The main postulate of goal theory is that the employee's goals are the predominant determinants of workplace behaviour. Trainers should encourage goal-setting behaviour to motivate the VDP; the professional development portfolio is a useful tool in this respect. Goal theory works well in practice provided that the goals are realistic and achievable.

Goals set jointly are more likely to be achieved and it has been shown that people who set (themselves) difficult goals invariably perform better. The convenient catch-all approach, which encourages VDPs to 'do the best you can', without setting goals is woefully inadequate.

3 *Expectancy theory*

The expectancy theory (VH Vroom) suggests that motivation is a function of:

• what the employee wants to happen
• level of performance in relation to effort
• level of reward in relation to performance
• the strength of belief that a particular desired outcome will satisfy his/her needs.

Anticipation of expected events is usually based on past experience, but in many cases the VDP will not have any past experience of practice. The theory suggests that if there is no opportunity to rely on past experience, as is often the case in vocational training, then motivation levels are reduced.

One of the frequently voiced concerns amongst trainers is that the VDP's salary needs are not linked to performance. This is deemed by many to be a limiting factor as far as motivation is concerned and would appear to accord with Vroom's expectancy theory. The other view is that a salary–performance link would somehow undermine the educational purpose of the year. The debate continues.

It should be noted that trainers are not permitted to offer incentive payments in relation to performance targets.

The reader is referred to widely available texts on the work of Maslow and Herzberg for more details on the subject.

Professional

Poor performance can result from a failure to exercise skills specific to dentistry but also from a range of generic skills that include communication skills and problem solving. It is interesting to note that, in its proposals for the future of postgraduate dental training, SCOPME noted that 'Generic

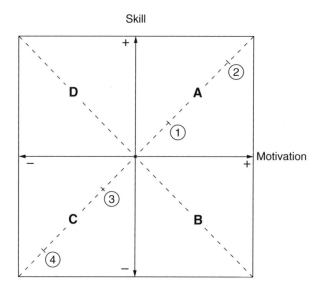

Figure 15.2 The skill-motivation matrix.

skills should be written into the aims of a course and the opportunities for their development made explicit to trainees ...' (SCOPME, 1999).

The reasons for poor performance are not always easily identifiable. Poor performance is an umbrella term for a host of factors, most of which can be categorised in relation to skills and motivation. A skill-motivation matrix is one way of considering the issues (Figure 15.2).

In this approach, the performance of the VDP can be categorised in any one of four domains, which are characterised by the degree of skill and motivation attributed to them. Within each domain, performance can vary according to the position occupied by the VDP on the dotted line of each domain.

For example, a VDP who possesses good clinical skills and is well motivated can occupy any position on the dotted line in domain A. An exceptional performer would occupy position 2, but a less able (but still competent) individual may occupy position 1 on the line.

VDPs who have the motivation but lack technical and/or generic skills would be assigned to category B. These individuals will require opportunities to observe and practise to overcome the skill deficit. Category C is for those who have poor motivation and poor skills, and those with good skills but poor motivation would be represented in category D.

In reality, the practising circumstances of poorly performing VDPs are rarely this simple, but this model does at least help to understand the fundamental categories. Once the category of poor performance has been identified, the process of remedying the situation is very much easier.

A VDP who lacks a particular skill but who is motivated to acquire it is easy to deal with, but individuals who fall into the peripheral zone of domain C can be more difficult to manage. In this case, there may be serious concerns about professional competency. The seriousness of this dilemma is reflected in the fact that the challenge of dealing with the so-called 'dysfunctional VDP' (who probably occupies position 4 in domain C) has been debated at the highest level in VT circles. Someone who occupies position 3 in this domain can be motivated by the role model facet of the trainer–VDP relationship and also by peer group influence.

The key processes in tackling poor performance rely firstly on recognition of the problem and then on its acceptance. The next step is to take responsibility for dealing with it, identifying the range of options and then deciding on which solution to implement.

The role of the trainer is to help the VDP identify the barriers to achievement and then help to overcome them.

Organisational

Organisational barriers arise from:

- time and financial pressures
- training bias
- staff expectations
- poor communication.

Time and financial pressures
Poor time management (which includes allowing too much time for procedures as well as too little) will have an adverse effect on work output. Financial measures of performance should not be a priority in the early part of the year, however, they are an important and integral part of general dental practice and the business of dentistry to which VDPs must be exposed.

Training bias
This is a view that the old tried and tested methods are best and that training should be carried out in the same way as it has been before. Inexperienced trainers sometimes make the mistake of thinking that VT is an extension of undergraduate teaching and will try to replicate the way they were taught themselves. Experienced trainers can make the mistake of believing that all they have to do is repeat what they did with their last VDP and everything will be alright. The needs of every VDP are different. There will, of course, be many similarities in the training schedule, but the pace, content and priorities will differ from year to year.

Staff expectations

Team members need to be fully briefed by trainers about aspects of vocational training in general dental practice, particularly if the practice has not participated in a VT scheme before. If their expectations of performance reflect their experiences in working with established practitioners, then there is the potential for conflict.

Poor communication

Communication and discussion of issues relevant to the practice should involve the VDP. There is a tendency sometimes to disregard the opinions of less experienced colleagues when it comes to matters of practice management. This can mean that decisions are taken and policies made without everyone in the team being aware of them. No wonder that some VDPs occasionally complain of alienation and inadequacy, which can dent their confidence and self-image. The remedy is to involve them in practice meetings and related social events.

If they are not involved, how can they be expected to contribute to organisational progress? If they are not valued, then why should they value the practice and the opportunities it has to offer?

Environmental

There is little doubt that social, economic and political factors influence trends in general dental practice. Many of these will impact on the business aspects of dentistry, which force practitioners to make certain changes to the way the practice is run. Economic constraints in any business or industry limit choice and options and can have a deleterious effect on quality.

Many despair at the thought of trying to meet the challenges of dental practice and not all would want to try. Faced with what many see as an impossible situation, a number of excellent training practices have been lost from the VT pool because the trainers no longer meet the eligibility criteria as far as their level of NHS commitment is concerned.

Stress-related issues

Stress is the physiological, emotional and psychological response that results from the VDP's interaction with the environment.

The relationship between stress and performance is shown in Figure 15.3. There is a level of stress that enhances performance, but the rela-

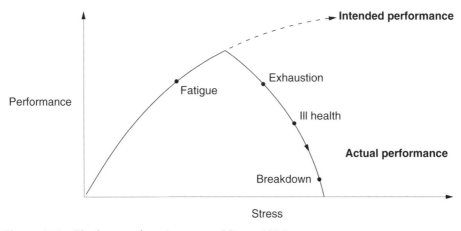

Figure 15.3 The human function curve (Nixon, 1976).

tionship soon falters when excessive stress levels result in decreased performance and eventual ill health.

The demands of practice management are second only to the clinical pressures of modern dentistry. The drive towards quality in all spheres of clinical and managerial practice places all dentists under considerable stress. Stress affects performance and undermines an individual's ability to cope with the rigours of daily practice.

Stress amongst dentists has been perceived as a problem for the profession for over 20 years. Numerous studies have been undertaken and identify the dental profession as a particularly stressful occupation. In surveys carried out amongst VDPs, the vast majority of VDPs either *agreed* or *strongly agreed* with the statement, 'all in all, I feel that I am under a lot of stress at work'.

The signs of stress fall into three categories (Table 15.1):

1 *physical signs*, which include perspiration, fatigue, muscular pain
2 *emotional symptoms*, which include rapid mood changes, overreaction to minor problems, irritability and lack of concentration
3 *behavioural disturbances*, which include indecision, increased alcohol intake, poor performance, lowered quality of work, disturbed sleep pattern.

Stress management

The management of stress should be a high priority for the VDP and the trainer and begins with an understanding of the general and more specific causes.

Table 15.1 The signs of stress

Physical signs	Emotional symptoms	Behavioural disturbances
• perspiration	• rapid mood changes	• indecision
• indigestion	• overreaction to minor	• increased rate of error
• palpitations	problems	• increased alcohol intake
• muscle fatigue leading	• irritability	• lowered quality of work
to muscular pain	• anxiety	• disturbed sleep pattern
• neck pains	• a lack of concentration	• overeating
• headaches		

General causes
The general causes of stress include:

- feelings of personal or professional inadequacy
- frustration at work
- lack of communication with peers and colleagues
- poor interpersonal relationships
- overwork
- quantitative overload
- qualitative overload
- poor self-image
- low self-esteem.

Some of these causes, for example poor self-image or frustration, may reflect other root causes.

Specific causes
VT surveys have identified the five most common stressors amongst VDPs to be (Rattan, 1992):

- patient management
- staff management
- business management
- maintaining clinical standards
- time pressures.

Early recognition of symptoms remains an important aspect in stress management. The effects of prolonged exposure to stress are identifiable and this is often the first indication that something is wrong. The absolute measurement of stressors remains difficult, mainly because it is subjective. Particular situations may induce the condition in one individual but may provoke an entirely different response in another.

The perception of the situation has important implications in stress management. Altering the perceptions can be an important weapon in coping with a stressful situation. Trainers should aim to help VDPs see things in perspective and learn to look at things in a different way.

Time should be set aside to discuss potential problems before they escalate into more serious concerns.

Strategies for stress management can be broken down into three areas:

Personal
Coping strategies include:

- making time for leisure and recreation
- spending time with family and friends
- improving physical fitness
- setting realistic goals
- avoiding conflict.

Professional
Coping strategies relating to professional issues include:

- managing change effectively
- delegating effectively
- improving practice systems and procedures
- setting realistic goals and objectives
- avoiding conflict
- predetermining workload
- preventing overload
- avoiding overcommitment.

The last three are all part of effective time management.

Work environment
The work environment should be carefully studied and designed to reduce stress potential. This can often be achieved with minimal intervention. For example, a review of the workplace may involve the following actions:

- alter physical layout for optimum ergonomics
- check heating and lighting levels
- spread the burden of responsibility
- manage time effectively
- improve management systems
- observe health and safety standards

- carry out repairs promptly
- allow time to handle paperwork.

Other coping strategies include a variety of relaxation techniques that are rapidly gaining favour. These include autogenic training, physical activity, breathing exercises and biofeedback techniques.

Stress surveys have identified some general coping strategies, which are listed below in order of frequency:

1 change lifestyle habits to build stress resistance
2 compartmentalise home and work life
3 take regular exercise
4 talk it through on the job with peers
5 physical withdrawal from a stress-provoking situation
6 substitution – change to an engrossing but non-work-related activity
7 talk it through with spouse
8 review workload
9 analyse situation and alter strategy
10 change to different work task – the so-called 're-direction' strategy.

Whilst it is neither possible nor desirable to eliminate all the causes of stress, it is important to recognise it and to deal with when it occurs. One way to do this is to use a simple grid such as that shown in Table 15.2.

A group of VDPs who recently completed this questionnaire ranked their responses in the following order:

1 take a complete break
2 seek discussion with friends and colleagues
3 passive relaxation
4 use laughter
5 feel anger towards patients/the system
6 avoid stressful situations
7 manage time better
8 take more exercise
9 drink more alcohol
10 overeat
11 delegate tasks
12 be irritable
13 drive fast
14 seek counselling.

Trainers may wish to compare these responses with those of their VDP or the current peer group.

Table 15.2   Stress Response Questionnaire (reproduced with permission from Chambers, 1999)

Response to stress	Never or seldom	Sometimes	Often	Ranking
Seek discussion with colleagues or friends				
Drive at high speed				
Overeat				
Delegate tasks to practice staff				
Passive relaxation, e.g. TV, relaxation tape				
Have a complete break when not on duty				
Seek counselling				
Be irritable with colleagues or patients				
Drink more alcohol				
Take more exercise				
Manage time better				
Avoid stressful situations				
Feel anger towards patients or colleagues or the system				
Use laughter or jokes				
Other:				
Other:				

Other responses might be to reduce caffeine/coffee, play music, get a pet, take up a new hobby, sleep, pray, yoga.

Compare the answers with those of a group of VDPs who completed this questionnaire.

CHAPTER 16

Common concerns

Four surveys involving a number of London-based schemes were undertaken over a consecutive three-year period in an attempt to identify the most frequently voiced concerns amongst trainers and VDPs. In each year, representatives from each group were asked for suggestions on how these concerns might be addressed.

The purpose was to try and identify concerns and give trainers and VDPs the solutions at the outset to lower the potential for conflict early in the training year. The results were used as part of the study day induction course for trainers and VDPs.

This chapter summarises the concerns that were consistently raised and proposed solutions.

Many of the concerns are real-life scenarios that experienced trainers have encountered on many occasions. The solutions are not prescriptive, but they are a true and accurate reflection of the collective views of experienced trainers.

Readers may have their own views on how best to approach some of the potential problems and readers new to VT may find the views of peers helpful.

Trainers' concerns

1   *I do not have enough time to train*
    Make time in your schedule and diary to accommodate your VDP's needs. This is particularly important in the early stages of training where there may be more need for hands-on help. Refer to the trainers' handbook for a suggested timetable for the early weeks of training.

    Plan your appointment book to allow some time at the end of the day to review the VDP's day, particularly in the early stages of training. A good start will pay dividends later in the year. Do not look at this time as 'lost earnings', rather as an investment for a trouble-free training year. Experienced trainers confirm that this approach can prevent problems later.

2 *I am concerned whether the VDP will fit in to my existing team*
Introduce your VDP to the rest of the team. Do this early and don't
rush it. Make sure everyone has time to get to know a little bit about
each other.

Involve the VDP in staff meetings and encourage them in decision-
making processes and ask them for their views if you plan to make
some changes in the practice. This will also help with motivating
them.

Make it clear to the staff that the VDP is a qualified dentist.

3 *My VDP seems to be taking excessive sick leave*
Differentiate between genuine illness and contrived conditions.

Keep accurate records and discuss the situation with your VDP in
a non-confrontational way and in private. There may be a more
serious underlying problem and some counselling may be needed.
Explain the disruption it causes to practice routine and the extra
stress it places on staff when patients have to be cancelled at short
notice.

If you are fair with your VDP then hopefully he or she will be fair
to you. Excessive sick leave is sometimes one way that an aggrieved
employee feels they can 'can get back at you' for any injustices they
feel may have occurred.

4 *My VDP is not motivated*
Try to identify the cause of lack of motivation. Are there any personal
or domestic factors that may be causing the VDP excessive stress. Try
to discuss these. There have to be good communication channels
between both parties if problems like this arise and need to be
resolved.

Discuss with your VDP what they feel about dental practice. Look
for ways of making the training more appropriate to the needs of your
VDP. It may be that the VDP's patients do not offer him or her a
variety of work (there have been some cases where VDPs have been
seeing the 'rejects' from everyone else in the practice, or a dispropor-
tionate number of children). Try to create this variety.

Involve the VDP more in the day-to-day running of the practice.
Try to delegate some of the responsibilities to make them feel more
involved and a part of the team. Offer encouragement and praise
when it is indicated. Remember the old adage 'praise in public but
criticise in private'.

5 *My VDP is slow with his or her paperwork*
Explain the importance of the forms and why it is necessary to

complete and despatch them within a reasonable time of completion of treatment. If necessary, refer to the NHS Rules and Regulations to back up what you say. Explain the importance of prompt despatch in terms of cash flow to the practice. How would the VDP feel if their pay cheque were delayed at the end of the month?

Prompt despatch of approvals, etc. is necessary to provide a good standard of service to patients – remind them of their ethical obligations to the patients.

6   *My VDP has difficulties in treatment planning*
If this occurs in the early stages of training, it could be that there are too many complex cases for the VDP to treat too quickly. The introduction to general practice should be gradual and at a measured pace.

Arrange for joint treatment planning sessions and joint consultation appointments for cases so that the VDP is able to see how his or her trainer copes with potentially complex treatment plans.

Make treatment planning a subject for discussion in one or more tutorials.

7   *My VDP seems to get a lot of failed appointments and/or incomplete treatment cases*
Approach this problem with caution and do not jump to conclusions. Assess the percentage of patients that fail or do not complete treatment and compare this with the others in the practice. This information can be easily obtained from the spreadsheets you have been provided with.

Analyse the type of patients that the VDP is seeing. Are they mostly new patients, or poorly-motivated patients? This may account for part of the problem.

If the patients are existing patients who have previously had a good record of attendance and have suddenly started to miss appointments or fail to return, then your apprehensions may be well-founded, in which case you should sit in with the VDP during his or her clinical sessions and see if you can identify what weaknesses surface. There may be problems with clinical knowledge, practical skills or attitude. Focus the content of your training schedule on the identifiable weaknesses and speak with your scheme adviser so that the relevant areas can be explored on the study days. Quite often an attitude change can be brought about by peer group pressure.

Ask the VDP for his or her opinion on the problem.

Consult with your receptionist and/or the VDP's DSA to see if any comments are being made to them by patients.

As a last resort you may wish to contact the patients yourself to hear their views. It was generally felt that this was impractical and very difficult to do, but that it was, nevertheless, an option. It may be easier to carry out an 'exit survey' of patients who have visited the VDP.

When the cause has been identified, discuss it with your VDP. There may be difficulties in communication between him or her and the patients, or clinical weaknesses, etc. Identify the problem and try and overcome it in tutorials or in joint working sessions.

8   *My VDP isn't working hard enough*
First, ask yourself what you expect of them, and compare your expectations with other trainers. Be realistic in your expectations and remember that you cannot expect the same performances that you would expect from an associate.

Speak to your course organiser for another view on the subject.

Keep your worksheets up to date so that you can assess clinical output objectively and compare it with others on the course or others from previous years. Your VT adviser will also be able to give you some idea of your VDP's performance relative to other members of the group.

9   *My VDP is losing me money*
See solutions to (8) above.

Remember also to compare 'like for like' and to check how patients' list size can cause anomalies when comparing schedules fees. It has been known for some trainers to compare schedule gross fees and not take list sizes into account, which enhance gross fees through continuing care and capitation payments.

Remember to take into account that there will be at least another three schedules to come after the training year has finished.

Sit in with the VDP during clinical sessions, see how they are working and make suggestions to them (in private) as to how they might improve their efficiency without compromising their clinical standards.

Use the professional development portfolio as a tool to help identify possible causes. The work analysis spreadsheets are useful to assess possible areas of weakness and equate work output with time taken and gross fees received. Discuss the findings with your VDP and compare your statistics with national trends.

Look at cost per estimate statistics from the schedules and compare them with the average for your practice and your Health Authority area. (Your most recent DPB practice profile will give you this information as a guide.) Discuss the findings with your VDP.

Remember that financial pressure in the early stages of training is inappropriate. Give VDPs a reasonable settling in period. The length of this will vary from individual to individual.

Look at the equipment in the surgery and ensure that everything is functioning. It has been known for VDPs to book longer sessions than necessary to allow time for autoclaving of handpieces, etc. between patients. If there are insufficient instruments, work progression may be halted.

Remember that the early months of VT are usually loss making (*see* Chapter 14).

10 *My VDP demands different materials and equipment*
Recent graduates do not always have the experience of the variety of dental materials and products available today. It is estimated that there are over 8000 lines stocked by the larger manufacturers and no one can be expected to be familiar with all of them. One of the common problems is that VDPs do not always appreciate that two products are very similar because they have become accustomed to remembering brand names. One way around the problem is to analyse what they are asking for and to see if you have an equivalent generic material in the practice.

If the VDPs persist on using a particular material, then give them the opportunity to discuss its merits with you. In short, they should convince you of the benefits and it is then up to you to consider the matter. Remember, they could be right!

VDPs' concerns

1 *I am afraid that I will be asked to use inferior materials*
Remember that dental materials have to conform to minimum standards so it is unlikely that you will be using materials of poor quality. However, as with all things in life, you can always buy something better. Discuss with your trainer what you would like to use and why, and what problems you are having with your existing materials. He or she may offer you some advice that will enable you to obtain better results with what you already have in the practice.

Make a case for purchase, and trainers have agreed to accede to reasonable requests. But remember that it is your responsibility to be economical with use, avoid wastage and be sure to use up what you have asked for.

2 *I will not be allowed to use the materials I want*
Do not let this become an issue. Accept that it is impossible for train-

ers to buy you everything you want; they have to exercise some degree of budgetary control over stock as a way of curbing expenditure. However, this does not mean that you should not be able to make reasonable requests and meet with some success, at least. It is a matter of give and take.

3 *I am concerned that I will not be allowed enough time for clinical procedures*
During the early stages of your training, the trainers accept that you need more time for clinical procedures than will the experienced practitioner. Make sure that your nurse and the receptionist know about this so that they are fully in the picture about how much time you require.

As you develop your clinical skills and become more practised at executing them, your procedure times should contract; your trainers will expect this from you as the year progresses.

4 *I am worried about treating and getting on with difficult patients*
First, remember that the handling of difficult patients is part of daily practice. Everyone has difficult patients and you are not alone in expressing this reservation.

Discuss individual situations with your trainer and seek his or her guidance at all times. Ask if you can sit in on clinical sessions to see how your trainer copes with difficult patients.

Remember that you are a professional person; maintain your professional demeanour and professional courtesy at all times. This can help to defuse the threat.

Try to find out why patients are being difficult. It may be that they are kept waiting too long before they are seen – in which case the underlying problem is not necessarily the patient but the fact that you are running late – for which there may be a perfectly legitimate reason. Discuss with your trainer and your colleagues on the course how they would handle the situation.

5 *I am concerned that I will need to lower my standards of practice because of time pressure*
Trainers have agreed that they would not wish you to lower your standards to unacceptable levels. Your aim should be to work efficiently to your standards and to become skilful at managing your time efficiently. It is possible to perform good dentistry efficiently.

6 *I am concerned about the standards of infection control*
Discuss your reservations with your trainer.

Compare your methods for cross-infection control with the

methods used in other surgeries and practices by discussing the problem with your peers on the scheme. Present your findings to your trainer in an objective rather than emotive fashion.

The whole of the dental profession is concerned about cross-infection controls and your trainers will welcome practical suggestions as to how this may be improved.

7 *What if I am not given clinical freedom?*

The majority of trainers have indicated on their application form that they provide a full range of NHS work for you. They have also confirmed this intention at the course, so you should have an opportunity to provide a variety of work within the NHS.

Within reason, they are agreeable for you to have clinical freedom. However, if your prescribing pattern is significantly different from the other dentists in the practice or other dentists in the area then it is not unreasonable that you and your trainer should discuss this and try and work out why this should be. To this extent, trainers are required to monitor and oversee your clinical activity.

Also remember that there will be restrictions on your clinical freedom imposed by the NHS rules and regulations. You are required to work within these

8 *Will I be under excessive time pressure?*

You should have a great deal of flexibility in how much time you require at the early stages of your training and should not be under any pressure.

However, as your year progresses and your clinical experience increases, it is important that you appreciate that efficiency is important. You should monitor this yourself and see how you are progressing. A great deal of time is often wasted during a clinical session and you should aim to endeavour to identify wastage and strive to eliminate it. This will enable you to carry out your clinical work to the same standard but in less time. Efficient working practices do not necessarily mean lowered standards.

9 *I am not receiving any/enough tutorials*

Your trainers are obliged by contract to provide one hour each week for tutorials. This time is part of your 28–35-hour contractual requirement. Therefore tutorials should be held during working time. Plan and book these in advance.

This obligation remains in force for the entire duration of the training year.

However, if you and your trainer both feel that an alternative schedule is better suited to both your needs, you may present your alternative to your scheme organiser for confirmation.

10 *I have heard that some people receive incentive payments in addition to their salary. Should I suggest this to my trainer?*
No. This is not permitted.

CHAPTER 17

Clinical governance

Clinical Governance (CG) is now an integral part of general dental practice. VDPs should be introduced to the principles of clinical governance from the outset of their training year. They should be aware of the different facets of clinical governance that apply to general dental practice (Figure 17.1).

The purpose of clinical governance is to encourage an approach to patient care that delivers:

- a focus on quality
- a commitment to finding ways of improving that quality
- a willingness to implement systems which evaluate outcomes.

In fact, when you think about it, it is what dentists in general practice do all the time. These are the foundations of running a successful dental practice. CG is concerned with ensuring that what is done in our practice

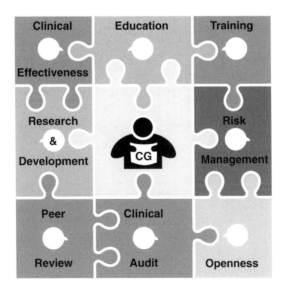

Figure 17.1   Elements of clinical governance in vocational training.

on a day-to-day basis is of quality and is underpinned by evidence. Because it is about finding ways do it better, it is adaptable to many aspects of vocational training.

If there is concern about the implications of CG, then that is more a reflection of perceptions than the reality of the situation. David Haslam, a GP and writer from Cambridgeshire, summed it up rather nicely when he wrote that 'the concept of clinical governance has become something as unwelcome as a dental check-up. We know that we have to do it, we know that it is really for the best, but we simply cannot dig deep and find any enthusiasm for the process' (Chambers and Wakley, 2000).

Background

The driving force behind clinical governance was the 1997 White Paper, *The New NHS: modern, dependable* (Department of Health, 1997).

There are ten so-called pillars of clinical governance (NHS Executive). This listing of them gives trainers a useful framework on which to build the clinical governance protocols in their practice. They are that:

1 quality improvement processes are in place and integrated with the quality programme for the practice as a whole
2 leadership skills are developed at clinical team level
3 evidence-based practice is in day-to-day use and has the infrastructure to support it
4 good practice, ideas and innovations are systematically disseminated within and outside the practice
5 clinical risk reduction programmes of a high standard are in place
6 adverse events are detected and openly investigated and the lessons learned are promptly applied
7 lessons for clinical practice are systematically learned from complaints made by patients
8 problems of poor clinical performance are recognised at an early stage and dealt with to prevent harm to patients
9 all professional development programmes reflect the principles of clinical governance
10 the quality of data gathered to monitor clinical care is itself of a high standard.

VT and clinical governance

Clinical governance was always intended to be organisation-based. It was first defined as

> *a framework through which NHS organisations are accountable for continuously improving the quality of their services and safeguarding high standards of care by creating an environment in which excellence in clinical care will flourish.*

A good place to start in VT is to encourage the VDP to carry out a clinical audit. Clinical audit/peer review was described as 'a central pillar of clinical governance' in the government's guidance document *Modernising NHS Dentistry: clinical audit and peer review in the GDS* (Department of Health, 2001).

Clinical audit

A Government White Paper, *Working for Patients* (Department of Health, 1989) defined audit as

> *the systematic critical analysis of the quality of medical care, including the procedures used for diagnosis and treatment, the use of resources and the resulting outcome and quality of life for the patient.*

The definition, however, gives little guidance on purpose and process. An extended definition could add that clinical audit is a process of self- and peer-evaluation of the quality of dental care by objective means to assess and improve the quality of patient care.

VDPs will understand that practices must monitor and evaluate the quality of service provided for patients. By way of comparison, the purpose of quality control in other industries is to reduce the incidence of faulty goods reaching the market place and thereby contaminating the reputation of the business.

The audit cycle

The three components of audit are:

* purpose
* methodology
* subject matter.

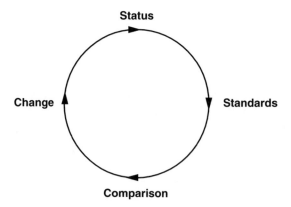

Figure 17.2 The audit cycle.

All audit activity is cyclical. It is based on four key activities (Figure 17.2).

The starting point in this cycle is a review of current performance. The standards against which VDP performance is to be measured should be agreed prior to the comparative analysis.

Changes should then be introduced to bridge the gap between actual and agreed performance levels. The professional development portfolio can be used to record the outcome of the audit and this, in turn, can be used to devise the action plan for future development and help to define learning goals.

Setting standards and guidelines

It may be helpful to define the various terms used in audit and monitoring as they are sometimes used interchangeably and therefore incorrectly.

Guidelines are systematically developed statements to assist practitioner and patient decisions about appropriate healthcare for specific clinical circumstances (Field and Lohr, 1990).

Criteria are systematically developed statements that can be used to assess the appropriateness of specific healthcare decisions, services and outcomes (Field and Lohr, 1990).

An audit protocol is a comprehensive set of criteria for a single clinical condition or aspect of organisation

A standard reflects the percentage of events that should comply with the criterion (Baker and Fraser, 1995).

An indicator is a measurable element of practice performance for which there is evidence or consensus that it can be used to assess quality, and hence change in quality, of care provided (Lawrence and Olesen, 1997).

The level of performance expected from the VDP will be determined by internally agreed criteria between trainer and VDP and by externally set standards.

Internally agreed criteria are influenced by:

- clinical interests
- the trainer's previous experiences of VT
- the incidence of patient complaints
- SWOT analysis
- The VDP's undergraduate influences
- The VDP's peer group.

In the widest sense, internally agreed criteria include those put forward by the profession for its members. These should be known, discussed and agreed with the VDP.

Externally set criteria are usually promoted from institutions, for example Government departments. Sometimes, these criteria can be rigid and inflexible and may be open to local interpretation.

Audit relies on a problem-solving approach, which should now be very familiar to readers. The problem-solving loop in Figure 17.3 shows the key steps in the process.

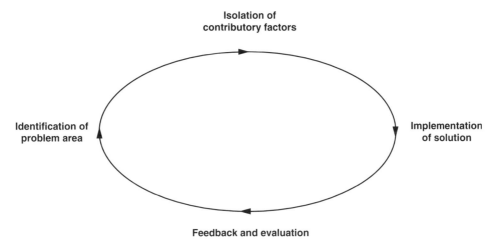

Figure 17.3 The problem-solving model.

Choosing topics

The choice of topic is a matter for the individual practice or practitioner. Broadly speaking, topics may be selected on the basis of:

- personal experience
- literature reviews
- identifiable weaknesses in the practice
- review of clinical records and radiographs
- current topics of interest
- VDP's perceived needs.

There are many areas of practice that merit further investigation, but the dentist will be limited by:

- clinical importance
- cost
- practicality
- ease of data collection and information gathering
- ease of measurement against standards.

Broad-based thinking facilitates the design of the audit process. At this stage of the process, the topic can be broad, but remember that the breadth of the subject matter complicates the evaluative functions in the cycle. Once the format and general outline of the audit programme has been determined, the subject matter should be pruned and the cyclical activities modified to suit.

Knowing where you are is always a good place to start. From status evaluation, the next stage is to study current standards. Attempts to set standards in an objective way have, perhaps unjustly, been met with considerable suspicion in the past. It is almost ten years since the publication of the Self-Assessment Manual for Standards (SAMS).

The low-key reception granted to SAMS can be attributed to its perceived purpose (as a stick with which to beat GDPs) and demonstrated that set targets and standards are often perceived as a threat unless there is active involvement of all parties. It is important for trainers therefore to make sure that VDPs are 'on board' with the concept before embarking on this process.

Resources

Trainers have access to data from a number of sources. These include:

- case reviews
- incidence occurrences
- adverse events
- criterion-based directives
- direct observation.

Case reviews are a simple but effective method of gathering information. The trainer and VDP can discuss case selection. Random selection of clinical records can be useful, but remember that it is non-specific. It may be more appropriate to select cases based on the needs of the VDP; random selections can be used again later in the training year.

In targeted cases, there has to be a reliable method of retrieving only those patient records that relate to the subject under audit. This is achievable if the practice is computerised and can access records by treatment type, or if the subject under review is common to many patients, say intra-oral radiographs, but it may be more difficult to locate relevant notes in other cases.

Another approach to case studies is the analysis of adverse occurrences. If this approach appears somewhat limited in its scope for audit purposes, it is worth remembering that it is suggested that the incidence of adverse occurrences in medicine is believed to be in the region of 20%.

Occurrence screening is another useful tool. Consider, for example, pain following root canal therapy. This particular outcome can be used as part of an 'occurrence screening' method of data collection. Occurrence screening involves a serial review of a number of patients undergoing a particular treatment. Cases are screened and outcomes of treatment are evaluated against predetermined criteria and standards. The results are analysed to identify trends or common occurrences which, if they fall short of agreed standards, should lead to revisions in clinical techniques and case management to improve the quality of future care.

In a criterion-based audit, a series of simple questions that can be answered by a 'yes' or 'no' are asked about the way treatment is carried out. The criteria can be the same as those used to set standards and can be sought from the same sources.

For example, in the case of a chromium-cobalt partial denture, the criterion-based questions would include: 'Was a special tray used?', 'Was the denture designed?', 'Were rest seats and guide planes prepared?'.

Another approach to audit relies on the day-to-day observations of what takes place in the VDP's surgery. Observational methods are very suitable for auditing generic skills like patient management, communication skills and consultation skills. They can also be used to audit procedures such as infection control. Infection control also lends itself to a criterion-based appraisal. Observation tools include:

• video recordings
• monitoring patient management, e.g. waiting times
• exit questionnaires for patients
• simulations.

Video is widely used in medical practice as a useful tool for analysing the style and effectiveness of consultations, but is less popular in dental practice. Exit questionnaires may be used to obtain information from patients about communication skills, general perceptions about the quality of service at the practice, and so on. The questions to ask on exit questionnaires should adhere closely to Shaw's criterion-based guidelines (Shaw, 1990).

Simulation, or asking the 'What if?' question, is a useful way of observing procedures that are infrequent and where real-life rehearsal is not possible. CPR training is a good example.

An audit-based approach to training can only be valuable if there are demonstrable and positive changes in the VDP's performance.

This will be influenced by a number of factors, which include:

• local guidelines
• national guidelines
• feedback from the trainer and other team members
• disciplinary matters
• peer group influences
• teaching on the course study days
• research and development in the supporting industries.

The feedback loop is important and is the backbone of effective training. Feedback can be active where it involves the trainer, other practising colleagues, VT group discussions and peer review. It is said to be passive when statistical data and trends are made available to VDPs from local or national sources. One example of this would be the quarterly Dental Practice Board profiles, which are now made available to trainers, although it should be noted that the early profiles will not give a true and accurate picture of the pattern of clinical activity. This is because the statistical data is based on treatment completions. Because less complex treatments are likely to be completed earlier, this will skew the statistics.

Reports of disciplinary proceedings provide a wider feedback mechanism and encourage change by example, particularly if there is a punitive outcome. Trainers can use the annual reports and newsletters published by various professional organisations to draw attention to specific issues of topical interest. Examples include *BDA News*, the *GDC Gazette* and annual reports from medico-legal organisations.

Risk management

The other key area identified in the consultation document *A First Class Service* identifies clinical risk reduction as an important aspect of clinical governance (Department of Health, 1998). There are three facets to this:

- risks to patients
- risks to practitioners
- risks to the practice.

The implementation of statutory regulations such as the Control of Substances Hazardous to Health (COSHH) Regulations and the Data Protection Act, and learning from patient complaints as well as clinical risk reduction protocols, like the use of a rubber dam during endodontic procedures, all contribute towards minimising risks to patients.

Immunisation against hepatitis B, the wearing of protective spectacles and correct working posture are all examples of ways of minimising risks to practitioners and staff.

Patient satisfaction surveys, a commitment to quality, a high standard of patient care and sound business policies are just some of the many everyday examples of reducing an organisation's exposure to risk.

The fundamental objectives of clinical risk management are to:

- identify the potential for failure at both an individual and organisational level
- collate and collect relevant records that relate to an adverse event with a medico-legal perspective in mind
- examine the facts relating to the incident to learn valuable lessons for the future.

Dealing with mistakes

Human beings make mistakes. There will be times during the year when VDPs will seek assistance from trainers to help them deal with less than ideal treatment outcomes.

Seldom is there a single factor that can be identified as the 'reason' for failure. It is usually due to a combination of individual and organisational factors.

Interestingly, Mr Justice Sheen's report into the tragic capsizing of the *Herald of Free Enterprise* in 1987 highlighted this by drawing attention to the subtle but real difference between *active human failures* and *latent human failures*. The member of the crew who failed to shut the bow doors provides an example of *active* failure, and the inadequate organisational polices (*latent* failures) created an environment in which active failures were more likely to arise.

A review of the literature suggests that failures or unsafe acts can be classified into errors and violations. The management of 'failure' is an important part of the trainer's role. Failure can be analysed on the basis of causation – it can be due to *attentional slippage* or to *mistakes*.

Attentional slippage is said to occur when there is an unintended deviation from what was intended. An example would be the extraction of the wrong tooth in a situation where the clinical notes indicated another tooth. But, in a situation where the wrong tooth was extracted due to incorrect diagnosis, the adverse outcome would be classified as a mistake. *Mistakes* can be rule-based or knowledge-based. In the former case, a clinician would encounter a familiar situation but applies the wrong solution. Knowledge-based mistakes are said to occur in situations where the level of training or knowledge is insufficient to consider a rule-based option.

If the prevention of unsafe acts is the desired outcome of a risk management strategy, then a review of the likelihood of such incidents seems a good place to start. Studies have been carried out with the aim of quantifying the probability of error – a probability of 1 reflecting absolute certainty. The studies have highlighted some obvious, some important and some interesting conclusions. For example, an individual carrying out a totally new task (perhaps with inadequate knowledge and/or ineffective training) has an error of 0.75 (possibly more depending how distant the task is from the present competencies). At the other end of the scale, a highly familiar task carried out by a competent and experienced practitioner carries an error probability of 0.0005.

Studies confirm that environmental and psychological factors affect error probability. Of these, some are particularly relevant to general practice and VT. These include:

- a high workload – sometimes referred to as quantitative overload
- inadequate knowledge and/or skill
- inadequate supervision where the performer lacks experience – particularly important in the early phase of vocational training
- a stressful working environment
- the ability to handle and manage change.

For example, inexperience (as opposed to lack of training) multiplies the probability of error by a factor of three. Unfamiliarity with a given task or situation produces a 17-fold increase in error probability. Time shortage raises the risk by a factor of 11. This is a particularly relevant finding in vocational training given the fact that time pressure is one of the most frequently voiced concerns by VDPs in the early months of training and that the teaching of efficient work methods is a high priority for many trainers.

An appraisal, however subjective, of these areas would be an integral part of risk management in a general practice environment and would be regarded as an essential part of a clinical governance programme in practice.

Situations also arise in practice where adverse events occur as a result of deviations from an accepted or regulatory code of practice. The GDS Regulations and the Statement of Dental Remuneration are examples of documents that set out the requirements for providing care and treatment under the NHS. An alleged breach of the terms of service or an inappropriate claim for payment would constitute a 'violation'. It is more difficult to make objective statements about violations, but there are some general observations about what factors promote violation tendencies. These include:

- poor supervision and control
- group norms condoning violations
- misperception of hazards
- a macho culture, which encourages risk taking
- low self-esteem
- perceived licence to bend the rules
- ambiguous rules.

It is important to bear these factors in mind because there is a tendency for some VDPs to take unnecessary risks of violation and a macho peer culture may tend to encourage this. It is not a welcome observation, but it would be imprudent to deny its existence.

Many violations reflect the risk-reward principle, and random checking of clinical records, both internally and by outside bodies, can help to limit the threat of widespread abuse.

Clinical effectiveness and evidence-based practice

These two terms are used interchangeably, but clinical effectiveness can be defined as 'a measure of the extent to which a particular intervention works' and evidence-based practice is 'the conscientious and judicious use of current best evidence in the management of clinical care for individual patients'.

In VT, the trainer's clinical experience and guidance will play a big part in the VDP's understanding and practice of evidence-based dentistry, but this experience must be supported by additional evidence because not all evidence is given the same weighting.

In the hierarchy, the strongest evidence comes from randomised, controlled clinical trials where two or more groups of patients are assigned to different treatment conditions according to random assignment or by chance, maximising the probability that groups are similar in signs and symptoms before treatment is commenced.

Next in the hierarchy are the uncontrolled clinical trials or comparative treatment outcome studies where two or more groups of patients are assigned to different treatment conditions according to any method other than random assignment.

The weakest evidence comes from case studies where small groups of patients are followed up prospectively after treatment is begun and then examined for improvement. There is a real danger that this category of evidence is allowed to dominate teaching in vocational training but, whilst nobody would argue against its value, it must be supplemented with information gleaned from one or both of the other evidence sectors.

Evidence-based care, then, offers a bridge between science/research and clinical practice and the following sequence can be applied in VT:

1   note the patient's complaint
2   define the clinical problem
3   identify the information required to resolve the problem
4   conduct a search of the available evidence
5   identify the clinical message
6   apply yourself to the patient's problem.

In some cases, the patient's problem will be acute and the VDP can only exercise point 4 by resorting to immediate advice from the trainer or seeking hands-on help. On other occasions, in the treatment planning of complex cases or other non-urgent clinical situations, trainers can extend the remit of point 4 to include a search of the literature, or a discussion with colleagues on the study course, and then undertake points 5 and 6 as a tutorial-based exercise.

The remaining aspects of clinical governance relate to the creation of a learning culture. Aspects of this have been covered elsewhere in this book.

CHAPTER 18

The end of the year

The end of the training year is a time for reflection for all those involved in VT. It marks the end of a 12-month training programme, and the beginning of the planning stage for the next year for VT advisers and those trainers who will have reapplied for approval.

The end-of-year review will include:

• trainer performance
• VDP performance
• exit evaluation of study course
• end-of-year interviews and certification.

Trainer performance

The VT adviser monitors trainer performance constantly throughout the training year. Records of attendance on the study course and trainers' meetings are kept and the views and opinions of the VDPs are noted.

Observations relating to in-practice tutorials, a willingness to provide help on demand and the provision of an adequate working environment with regards to equipment, materials, staffing and an adequate supply of patients all contribute to evaluating the trainer's performance during the year.

All records are confidential.

VDP performance

This also takes place throughout the training year using a variety of methods that have been discussed more fully in other sections of this book. The professional development portfolio is made available for inspection by the postgraduate dental dean at the end-of-year interviews.

Exit evaluation of the study course

Much of the evaluation of course content is undertaken on an on-going basis, but a reflective evaluation over the year is useful because it identifies particularly memorable study days. It is interesting to note that the perceived value of some sessions can vary at this stage from what they were when the presentation was first given. This is a clear indication that value and worth can only be accurately evaluated against the backdrop of individual experience.

End-of-year interviews and certification

End-of-year interviews take place on a one-to-one basis with the post-graduate dental dean. In some regions, VDPs are asked to complete a questionnaire prior to interview.

A certificate to confirm completion of vocational training is issued at the end of the year and will be required for the application of a VT number.

The transition from VDP to associate

If the VDP is staying on at the practice, agreement must be reached on a number of issues before contracts are agreed. Both parties will need to agree on:

- percentage remuneration/expense sharing arrangements
- how and when to transfer patient lists
- arrangements for remedial treatment in cases where original treatment was carried out under the VT contract number
- arrangements for completing patient treatment plans that commenced under VT arrangements but will be completed under an associate contract.

Remuneration is a matter for individual negotiation but most VDPs will expect a remuneration package that reflects market trends at the time.

The dental list can be transferred using form DTR 7, which is available from the Health Authority. Capitation and continuing care payments will then be automatically transferred by the DPB from the date of transfer on receipt of the DTR 7.

Patients who have not completed treatment will need to sign two FP17 forms – one to reflect the treatment provided under the VT contract number and the second to reflect the treatment provided under the associate number. The forms should be secured and sent for processing with a note to indicate that completion has taken place under a different contract. The DPB will adjust the patient charge contribution accordingly.

If the VDP leaves the practice and there is to be no replacement, the patient list reverts to the trainer.

It should be noted that reapproval of trainers is not an automatic process. Trainers who wish to be considered again for approval are required to complete an application form in the normal way.

VT number

At the end of the year, the majority of VDPs will embark on a career in general dental practice. An application has to be made to the Health Authority (in England and Wales), Health Board (in Scotland) or Area Board (in Northern Ireland) to join the dental list and, at the same time, the VDP should apply for a VT number. The forms to do this are available from the Health Authority. It is not possible to apply for a VT number without first submitting an application to join the dental list of a Health Authority. This procedure is still in place at the time of writing (August 2001), but given the imminent reorganisation of the NHS, the role of health authorities is likely to change in the near future. The process is summarised in Figure 18.1.

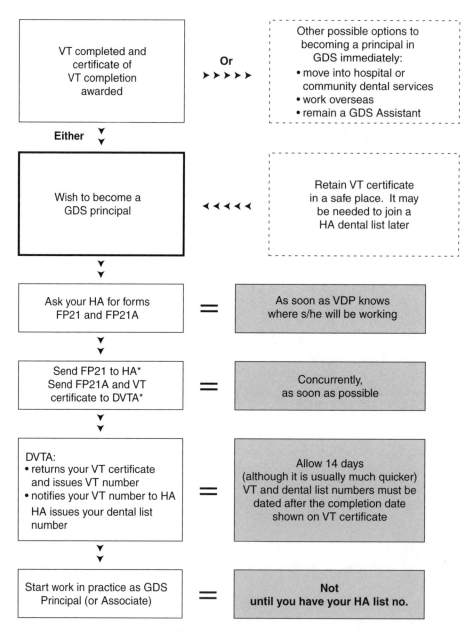

* Addresses as stated on forms FP21 and FP21A

Figure 18.1 Transition from VDP to Associate.

CHAPTER 19

General professional training

Vocational training for general dental practice has evolved in the last ten years to become an integral part of the professional career structure. It has remained as a one-year programme of study despite the fact that proposals for a two-year period of postgraduate training after qualification were first suggested as long ago as 1981 by the Dental Strategy Review Group.

The GDC Education Committee's *Statement on Vocational Training* (May 1987) advocated the same approach and this was further endorsed by the British Dental Association in the same year.

In 1995, the Chief Dental Officer's report drew attention to the fact that 'the feasibility of introducing a two-year period of general professional training' should be tested through pilot schemes, support for which was forthcoming in the Government White Paper *Primary Care: delivering the future* (Department of Health, 1996).

General professional training has been defined as 'the structured further development of knowledge, skills and attitudes common to all branches of the dental profession which will provide a basis for informed career choice and patient care'.

The Standing Committee on Postgraduate Medical and Education (SCOPME was disbanded in March 1999) published its findings in *The Early Years of Postgraduate Dental Training in England: an agenda for change* in February 1997 and made a number of recommendations. These were as follows.

- All organisations and groups within dentistry should examine the ways in which they communicate and collaborate to ensure that they do so in the most effective manner. This should be done with the help of outside experts if necessary.
- Organisations should re-examine the value of audit.
- The evaluation of innovation in education and training needs further work and relevant bodies should undertake this task.
- Those conducting the two-year pilot schemes in general professional training should consider undertaking comparative studies of the training arrangements in hospital and general dental practice.

- A steering committee for general professional training should be formed comprising representatives of all the stakeholders.
- The role of a 'core plus options' approach to postgraduate dental training should be examined further. Postgraduate dental deans should provide opportunities for consultants and other career grade staff to develop their roles as educators.
- Postgraduate dental deans should ensure that SCOPME's recommendations about formal educational opportunities apply to dental training.
- Time for training should be properly reflected in educational contracts between postgraduate deans, trusts and GDP trainers and in GDP and hospital trainers' job plans. It should be reflected in service contracts between purchasers and NHS trusts.
- Coherence in assessment is needed in the different health sectors during general professional training and further work is needed by experts in this area.
- All dental trainees should participate in appraisal.
- Training in health promotion and disease prevention should be given much higher priority.

These recommendations have influenced the continual development of postgraduate dental education in recent years. In particular, the notion that dentists should have some experience in primary and secondary care has been piloted in two-year GPT pilot schemes. The experimental schemes have been designed in one of two formats with some local variations.

1 A two-year programme with vocational training done on a full-time or part-time pro rata basis and secondary care training in either hospital and/or community services on a full-time or part-time pro rata basis.
2 The VT year is completed in the usual way and an optional second year is made available to develop elements of primary and secondary care further. It should be emphasised that this is not 'second year' VT as it is often misnamed and misunderstood.

The notion of 'flexibility' has been central to many experimental schemes and a one-year VT programme has been an integral part of many schemes. Trainers should inquire locally if they are interested in participating in any pilots.

CVT has stated that GPT remains a voluntary activity and will continue to do so 'until such good evidence exists that the appropriate structures, validity and costs warrant a national mandatory programme'.

Examples

The first pilot scheme was organised in the West Midlands; schemes in Scotland and in the Northern and Mersey deaneries followed. All four schemes were organised in different ways but shared the common goal of allowing trainees to experience primary and secondary care settings.

The key features of the West Midlands' model of GPT were incorporated in the three elements of the second year (after one year of VT in either the GDS or CDS). These were:

- half-time associateships in approved general dental practices or community clinics
- senior house officer appointments for five sessions in Birmingham Dental Hospital
- 15 core study days during this year.

A formal evaluation of the scheme concluded that 'participants of the GPT scheme operating in the West Midlands possessed greater confidence and more advanced clinical skills at the end of the two-year period of general professional training than at the end of their VT year'. The advantages of the two-year programme over the one-year option were noted in the report *Evaluation of GPT: West Midlands* (Musselbrook *et al.*, 1999) and were identified as:

- accelerated achievement of postgraduate qualifications in a supported environment
- creation of dynamic training environments
- better communication between the different branches of the dental service and the breakdown of artificial barriers between primary and secondary care
- fewer referrals to hospitals, and dentists with more advanced clinical skills
- dentists with more career options and greater adaptability
- dentists who can make informed career choices and are satisfied with the options they have chosen
- dentists with a greater commitment to continuing professional development and lifelong learning.

In Scotland, 16 trainees completed one year in general practice and two six-month blocks in the hospital and community services between 1996 and 1998. The scheme received widespread support from the GP trainees with 87% recording their support for training in all three service sectors (Plowman and Musselbrook, 2000).

The benefits of the scheme were deemed to include:

- an improved understanding of the referral system from all points of view
- better appreciation of the work of the CDS
- better communication between the different branches of the dental service and the breakdown of artificial barriers between primary and secondary care
- dentists with more advanced clinical skills, good generic skills, informed career options and greater adaptability.

The less popular aspects of this two-year programme were:

- the trainees found it onerous to complete the variety of record books they were requested to keep
- the six-month blocks led to some problems with continuity of patient care in the hospital and community services
- GPT trainers needed to maintain a higher level of input than was required on the established schemes and need more support.

The future of GPT

At the time of writing no firm decisions have been made about the future development of GPT. The evaluations of the pilot schemes have been encouraging and it remains to be seen whether two-year GPT will become a mandatory requirement. The GPT Liaison Group is presently looking into a number of schemes and is due to report its findings by the end of 2001.

In *Doctors and Dentists: the need for a process of review*, SCOPME put forward some proposals for the future organisation of training. It surmised from questionnaires that 'the large majority of all respondents agreed that a training programme should be planned to include optional training modules with a common core of training in both primary and secondary care', and noted that many respondents 'favoured a move towards training where dentists work as part of a healthcare team. Trainees should have the opportunity to train alongside other health professionals' (SCOPME, 1999).

CHAPTER 20

Dento-legal aspects of VT

The dento-legal aspects of VT may be considered under the following headings:

- contractual obligations
- NHS regulations
- dealing with complaints
- negligence
- ethics.

Contractual obligations

The law of Contract is concerned with 'agreements (which may be for goods or services) which are binding on the parties'.

The contractual obligations in VT fall into four groups:

1 There is an educational contract between the trainer and the deanery. This contract outlines the roles and responsibilities of being a trainer.
2 The contract between trainer and VDP is a one-year contract of employment.
3 The contract for the provision of general dental services. Although it is the VDP who will provide the services, the contract is between the trainer and the health authority because the VDP is an assistant working under the trainer's number. The contractual requirements are set out in the NHS Regulations (1992).
4 Deaneries also have an educational agreement between the VDP and Postgraduate Dean, which sets out the expectations for the educational side of the VT year.

NHS Regulations

The General Dental Services (GDS) Regulations are the main regulations governing the provision of primary dental care in general dental practice.

VDPs should be aware of these Regulations at the start of the training year, and, in particular:

- the definitions of the words used in the Regulations
- the structure of the arrangements
- the schedules for the Regulations.

One way to impart knowledge of the Regulations is to consider those that may be relevant to treatment planning issues and tutorial discussion topics. Regulations will be better understood when they are related to real-life experiences; straight reading of the rulebook is seldom effective.

VDPs should possess a copy of the Regulations, Terms of Service and the Statement of Dental Remuneration. They are not entitled to a free copy because of their status as 'assistants', but trainers are encouraged to let them have access to their copy.

Discussion should take place between trainer and VDP over how some of the better known regulations are interpreted and the consequences of breaching them. For example, the standard of care provided under the NHS is defined in paragraph 20(1)(a) on the Terms of Service (Schedule 1), which indicates that a dentist shall 'employ a proper degree of skill and attention'; and paragraph 20(2) which states that 'when providing general dental services a dentist shall not provide care and treatment in excess of that which is necessary to secure and maintain oral health'.

The Dental Practice Board (DPB) employs a large number of dental reference officers (DROs) whose primary role it is to maintain standards and carry out probity checks. Patients are selected, usually at random, for examination in cases where treatment has been sought by prior approval or where treatment has been completed.

If a patient of the VDP has been selected for examination, it is good practice to review the clinical records for that patient and to discuss aspects of treatment provided, or proposed treatment in the case of prior approval, with the VDP. If there are exceptional circumstances, then the observations should be sent to the DRO on the proforma provided for the purpose. Trainers should review the treatment plans submitted for approval to ensure that there is a sound basis for the proposals, particularly during the early months of training.

The DRO prepares a report after examination that is coded with a number and a suffix letter. The suffix summarises the findings of the examination. The meanings attached to the various letters are summarised in Box 20.1.

Codes L and M present few difficulties' but trainers and VDPs should seek the advice of their defence organisation before responding to a request from the DPB for observations in the case of reports coded R or S.

Box 20.1   DRO report suffices

L   Treatment (or proposed treatment) satisfactory

M   Minor degree of clinical disagreement with proposal, or oral
       health not secured and maintained, but reason not significant

R   Moderate disagreement with treatment proposals, or oral
       health not secured and maintained, for a significant reason

S   Major disagreement with proposed treatment, or oral
       health not secured and maintained for a reason of major
       significance

H   DRO unable to give a view (in cases of lack or unavailability
       of evidence)

If the DPB is not satisfied with the response and feels that there is a *de facto* breach of the Regulations, it may lodge a formal complaint to the Health Authority. It will be the trainer who will be the subject of further investigations and/or disciplinary action under these circumstances because of the contractual relationship in place.

Dealing with complaints

The National Health Service Regulation, para 31(a), Schedule 1 NHS (GDS) (Amendment) Regulations 1996 oblige a dentist to establish and operate a practice-based procedure to deal with complaints. The salient features of this procedure are:

- to nominate a person who should be responsible for receiving and investigating complaints
- to record all complaints
- to acknowledge complaints within three working days
- To respond within ten working days, or as soon as reasonably practical, giving a summary of the investigations and conclusions
- to keep records of complaints separate from the clinical records.

The Regulations apply to Health Authority contract holders. In the event of a complaint against the VDP, the responsibility of dealing with

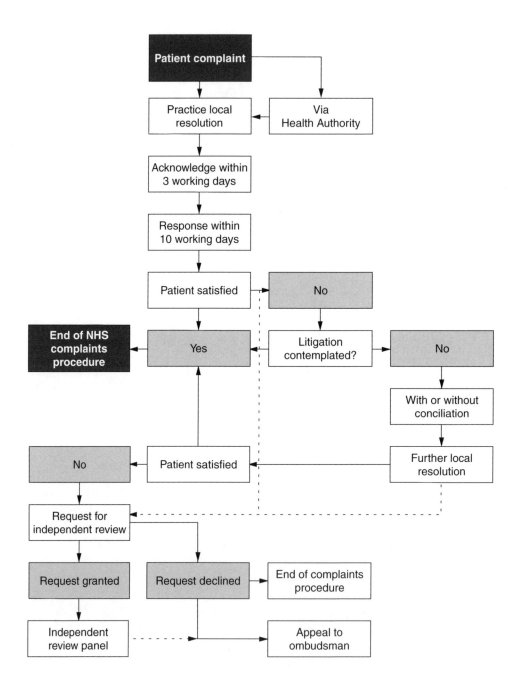

Figure 20.1 Complaints flowchart (reproduced by kind permission of Dental Protection Ltd).

the complaint rests with the trainer by virtue of (3) under Contractual obligations, *see* above.

The procedure is summarised in Figure 20.1.

Data from defence organisations confirms that the incidence of complaints against dentists in general dental practice is increasing at an alarming rate and there is some recent evidence to suggest that the incidence of complaints against VDPs is demonstrating a similar trend. There is also a positive correlation between poor communication and complaints incidence; trainers should stress the importance of effective communication with their VDP from the outset of the training year. A review of communication effectiveness should be a part of every practice's risk management strategy.

Negligence

Negligence may be defined as 'the omission to do something which a reasonable man, guided upon those considerations, which ordinarily regulate the conduct of human affairs, would do, or do something which a prudent and reasonable man would not do'.

Negligence is the breach of a legal duty to take care resulting in damage to the plaintiff which was not desired by the defendant. It connotes the concepts of duty, breach and damage thereby suffered by the person to whom the duty was owed. It has been said that it is 'not a state of mind, but a falling short of an objective standard of conduct'.

Any patient may contemplate an action to recover damages, but the burden of proof is generally on the plaintiff who must demonstrate that:

- the dentist owed a duty of care
- there was breach in that duty
- consequential damage was sustained – the nature of the damage is usually physical, but it may be psychological.

On occasions, the facts are self-evident and the maxim of *Res ipsa loquitur* (the thing speaks for itself) applies. Inhalation of a root canal instrument where no airway protection was used is one such example. In other cases, such as a fractured mandible during extraction, the courts have rejected pleas of *Res ipsa loquitur*.

The VDP is an employee of the trainer who may then be vicariously liable for the acts and omissions of the VDP and may be named in any proceedings that may arise. Vicarious liability is the liability that arises because of one person's relationship to another.

In a situation where a patient has been treated by the VDP, a separate action can, in theory, be brought against the trainer. Unless it can be shown that the VDP was being required to carry out a procedure beyond what could be reasonably expected to be within his or her competence, the courts will take the view that a registered practitioner must take responsibility for his or her actions.

However, in the situation where the trainer intervenes and offers hands-on help, say during a difficult surgical procedure, and the treatment then becomes the subject of an allegation of negligence, the trainer may also be directly implicated.

Under The Law Reform (Contributory Negligence) Act 1945, which introduced the concept of contributory negligence, a claim for damages may be reduced by an extent as the Court thinks fit having regard to the claimant's share in responsibility for the personal injury. Contributory negligence may arise when a patient fails to follow postoperative instructions, or reacts during treatment in a way that results in injury. For example, sudden movements during tooth preparation may result in a laceration of the cheek or tongue.

In a successful action, the Court may award monetary damages. The quantum of damages is the sum of *general damages*, the most common being compensation for pain and suffering, and *special damages*, which include the cost of remedial treatment, travel expenses and the loss of earnings.

Ethics

A VDP whose behaviour or actions bring the profession into disrepute (e.g. a criminal conviction) may face disciplinary proceedings at the General Dental Council. Trainers may find themselves party to such hearings if they have been directly or indirectly involved, or to give evidence. Many VT advisers incorporate a visit to observe disciplinary hearings at the General Dental Council in the study course. The visit often includes a seminar held at the headquarters of a defence organisation for part of the day where medico-legal aspects of dentistry can be explained in more detail.

References

Advisory Board in General Dental Practice, Faculty of Dental Surgery, Royal College of Surgeons (1991) *Self Assessment Manual for Standards (SAMS)*. ABGDP, FDS, RCS, London.

Aitken LA (1996) *Rating Scales and Checklists: evaluating behaviour, personality and attitudes*. Wiley, Chichester.

Baker R and Fraser RC (1995) Development of review criteria: linking guidelines and assessment of quality. *British Medical Journal*. **311**: 370–3.

Benner D (1984) *From Novice to Expert: excellence and power in clinical nursing practice*. Addison-Wesley, Menlo Park, CA.

Berne E (1969) *Games People Play*. Random House, London.

Berne E (1975) *What Do You Say After You Say Hello?* Corgi, London.

Black P and William D (1998) Inside the Black Box: raising standards through classroom assessment. *The Phi Delta Kappan*. **October**.

Bova B and Phillips R (1981) The significance of the mentor relationship in career development. *Journal of Adult Education*. **10**(1): 5–10.

British Dental Journal (1997) Experience of undergraduates from three London Dental Schools and trainers from the south east of England on interviews for vocational training in 1996. *British Dental Journal*. **183**: 284–8.

Brown GA (1982) Two days on explaining and lecturing. *Studies in Higher Education*. **2**: 93–104.

Brown S and McIntyre D (1993) *Making Sense of Teaching*. Open University Press, Buckingham.

Caird R and Ogden J (2001) Understanding the tutorial in general practice: towards the development of an assessment tool. *Education for General Practice*. **12**(1). 57–61.

Chambers R (1999) *Survival Skills for GPs*. Radcliffe Medical Press, Oxford.

Chambers R and Wakley G (2000) *Making Clinical Governance Work for You*. Radcliffe Medical Press, Oxford.

Chambers R and Wall D (2000) *Teaching Made Easy: a manual for health professionals*. Radcliffe Medical Press, Oxford.

Cowan J and Harding AG (1986) A logical model for curriculum development. *British J Educational Technology*. **17**: 103–9.

Cox K and Ewan C (1988) *The Medical Teacher*. Churchill Livingstone, Edinburgh.

Department of Health (1989) *Working for Patients*. Cm 555. The Stationery Office, London.

Department of Health (1992) *The National Health Service (General Dental Services) Regulations*. DoH, London.

Department of Health (1996) *Primary Care: delivering the future*. DoH, London.

Department of Health (1997) *The National Health Service Vocational Training of General Medical Practitioner Regulations*. DoH, London.

Department of Health (1997) *The New NHS: modern, dependable*. Cm 3807. The Stationery Office, London.

Department of Health (1998) *A First Class Service: quality in the new NHS*. DoH, London.

Department of Health (2001) *Modernising NHS Dentistry: implementing the NHS Plan*. DoH, London.

Dreyfus HL and Dreyfus SE (1984) *Mind Over Machine*. Macmillan/The Free Press, New York.

Eaton J (2001) Beyond the hype: on-line training. *Training Journal*. **March**: 32–5.

Editorial (1999) Being there. *The Dentist*. **May**: 6.

Field MJ and Lohr KN (eds) (1990) *Clinical Practice Guidelines: directions for a new program*. National Academy Press, Washington DC.

Guilbert J (1997) *Education Handbook for Health Personnel*. Offset Publication No. 35. WHO, Geneva.

Havelock P, Hasler J, Flew R *et al.* (1995) *Professional Education for General Practice*. Oxford University Press, Oxford.

Herzberg F (1959) *Two Factor Theory*. Publisher unknown.

Honey P and Mumford A (1986) *Using Your Learning Styles*. Honey Publications, Maidenhead.

Kinlaw DC (1997) *Coaching: winning strategies for individuals and teams*. Gower, London.

Kirkpatrick D (1959) Doctoral thesis. Unpublished.

Knowles MS (1975) *Self-directed Learning: a guide for learners and teachers*. Association Press, New York.

Kolb D *et al.* (1974) *Organisational Psychology: an experiential approach*. Prentice-Hall, London.

Lawrence M and Olesen F (1997) Equip Working Party on indicators of quality in health care. *European Journal of General Practice*. **3**: 103–8.

Levinson DJ (1979) *The Seasons of a Man's Life*. Ballantine Books, New York.

Maslow AH (1970) *Motivation and Personality* (2e). Harper & Row, London.

Middleton P and Field S (2001) *The GP Trainer's Handbook*. Radcliffe Medical Press, London.

Mossey P (1999) Training the trainers. *British Dental Journal*. **187**(2): 59.

Mowat H and Stewart S (1999) Using problem-based learning as part of general dental practice vocational training. *British Dental Journal*. **187**(2): 101–5.

Musselbrook K, Plowman L and Devine M (1999) *Evaluation of General Professional Training: West Midlands*. NHS Executive, University of Birmingham, NCCPED, Birmingham.

Nixon PGF (1976) Human Function Curve. *The Practitioner*.

Pereira Gray DJ (1979) *A System of Training for General Practice*. Royal College of General Practitioners, London.

Peters T and Waterman R (1988) *In Search of Excellence*. Macmillan, Basingstoke.

Plowman L and Musselbrook M (2000) An evaluation of general professional training for dentistry in Scotland. *British Dental Journal*. **188**(10): 563–7.

Prescott LE, McKinlay P and Rennie JS (2001) The development of an assessment system for dental vocational training and general professional training: a Scottish approach. *British Dental Journal*. **190**(1): 41–4.

Ralph JP, Mercer PE and Bailey H (2001) Does vocational training encourage continuing professional development? *British Dental Journal*. **191**(2): 91–4.

Rattan R (1992) *The Trainer's Handbook*. Committee on Vocational Training, London.

Rattan R (1998) *Illusions of Grandeur. The lecture: education or performance?* Diploma dissertation.

Riding R and Cheema I (1991) Cognitive styles: an overview and integration. *Educational Psychology*. **11**: 193–215.

Rogers A (1986) *Teaching Adults*. Open University Press, Milton Keynes.

Royal College of General Practitioners (1972) *The Future General Practitioner*. British Medical Association, London.

Samuel O (1990) What should trainees learn? *Postgraduate Education for General Practice*. **1**: 160-4.

Sanders J (1998) Mentoring and peer-supported learning. *Update*. **Nov**: 760–1.

Schon DA (1983) *The Reflective Practitioner*. Basic Books, New York.

SCOPME (1996) *Appraising Doctors and Dentists in Training*. SCOPME, London.

SCOPME (1997) *The Early Years of Postgraduate Dental Training in England: an agenda for change*. SCOPME, London.

SCOPME (1998) *Supporting Doctors and Dentists at Work: an enquiry into mentoring*. SCOPME, London.

SCOPME (1999) *A Strategy for Continuing Education and Professional Development for Hospital Doctors and Dentists.* SCOPME, London.

Shaw CD (1990) Criterion-based audit. *BMJ.* **300**: 649–51.

Skilbeck M (1975) School-based Curriculum Development and Teacher Education. Cited in M Mulholland (1988) *Curriculum Design and Development.* Centre of Medical Education, University of Dundee.

Tuckman BW (1965) Development sequences in small groups. *Psychological Bulletin.* **63**: 384-99.

Ward P (1997) *360 Degree Feedback.* Chartered Institute of Personnel Development's Developing Practice Series. CIPD, London.

Worthen B and Sanders J (1987) Objectives oriented evaluation approaches. In: *Educational Evaluation.* Longman, White Plains, NY.

Appendix 1
VDP survey

In April 2001, Lane and Bennett conducted an extensive survey of approximately 775 VDPs currently in post throughout the UK to gain an insight of their views on a wide-ranging number of professional issues. They received a 71% response rate to 18 questions. These highlight the current concerns and attitudes that this group of young professionals has to their career development. The results from this survey are reproduced here by kind permission of Andrew Lane and Adrian Bennett.

A fuller discussion of these results which includes further commentary from the respondents can be found on the website www.vtsurvey.com.

Prior to vocational training I envisaged a future in mainly NHS general dental services (GDS):

Strongly disagree	=	8%
Disagree	=	28%
Neither	=	23%
Agree	=	32%
Strongly agree	=	9%

My experiences as a VDP mean that I am now more likely to stay in the GDS:

Strongly disagree	=	10%
Disagree	=	27%
Neither	=	22%
Agree	=	33%
Strongly agree	=	7%

Recent government announcements on additional GDS funds have encouraged young practitioners to commit to a long-term future in the GDS:

Strongly disagree   =   15%
Disagree   =   50%
Neither   =   24%
Agree   =   10%
Strongly agree   =   1%

GDS regulations allow me to work to the standards I learned at dental school:

Strongly disagree   =   39%
Disagree   =   45%
Neither   =   7%
Agree   =   8%
Strongly agree   =   1%

GDS regulations encourage treatment planning that reflects the best interests of the patient:

Strongly disagree   =   21%
Disagree   =   43%
Neither   =   21%
Agree   =   14%
Strongly agree   =   1%

I am considering a future in a salaried position within a Dental Body Corporate:

Strongly disagree   =   19%
Disagree   =   29%
Neither   =   26%
Agree   =   24%
Strongly agree   =   2%

I am considering a future in private practice:

Strongly disagree   =   3%
Disagree   =   9%
Neither   =   18%
Agree   =   54%
Strongly agree   =   17%

I am considering a career within the hospital service:

Strongly disagree   =   19%
Disagree   =   28%
Neither   =   19%
Agree   =   27%
Strongly agree   =   7%

I am considering an academic career:

Strongly disagree   =   31%
Disagree   =   31%
Neither   =   18%
Agree   =   16%
Strongly agree   =   4%

I am considering a career in the community service:

Strongly disagree   =   38%
Disagree   =   32%
Neither   =   16%
Agree   =   12%
Strongly agree   =   2%

I am considering a career in a Dental Access Centre or PDS scheme:

Strongly disagree	=	33%
Disagree	=	39%
Neither	=	19%
Agree	=	9%
Strongly agree	=	1%

I wish to gain a postgraduate qualification:

Strongly disagree	=	1%
Disagree	=	3%
Neither	=	8%
Agree	=	39%
Strongly agree	=	49%

I hope to gain specialist status within 10 years:

Strongly disagree	=	8%
Disagree	=	18%
Neither	=	31%
Agree	=	22%
Strongly agree	=	21%

I would like to see a dental specialty of 'general dental practice':

Strongly disagree	=	2%
Disagree	=	13%
Neither	=	27%
Agree	=	42%
Strongly agree	=	15%

I believe that mandatory CPD is beneficial to the profession and public:

Strongly disagree	=	2%
Disagree	=	2%
Neither	=	9%
Agree	=	46%
Strongly agree	=	41%

The British Dental Association (BDA) works well for the interests of young GDPs:

Strongly disagree	=	2%
Disagree	=	9%
Neither	=	30%
Agree	=	48%
Strongly agree	=	11%

The BDA makes a good job of raising public awareness of dental issues:

Strongly disagree	=	5%
Disagree	=	16%
Neither	=	31%
Agree	=	41%
Strongly agree	=	6%

I believe there should be a core NHS dental service free at the point of delivery to all (e.g. relief of pain, extractions, dressings, acrylic dentures), with all other items available privately:

Strongly disagree	=	7%
Disagree	=	24%
Neither	=	19%
Agree	=	34%
Strongly agree	=	17%

Appendix 2
www.first-practice.com

www.first-practice.com has been designed primarily as a resource for dentists in the early stages of their practising career in general dental practice. It contains a wealth of useful information for trainers and VDPs. For example, trainers can download ideas for tutorials and other practice-based activities to facilitate their role. They can also discuss aspects of VT using the message boards.

VDPs can access information about topical issues in VT, trends in general practice and career opportunities once they finish VT. There is also a discussion forum, which allows VDPs from all parts of the country to communicate with each other.

Other areas on the site include information and ideas on all aspects of practice management, including marketing, business principles and CPD. Whilst these areas may not be of direct relevance during the VT year, they are nevertheless a useful resource for VDPs for the future. The site has been designed with this continuum in mind.

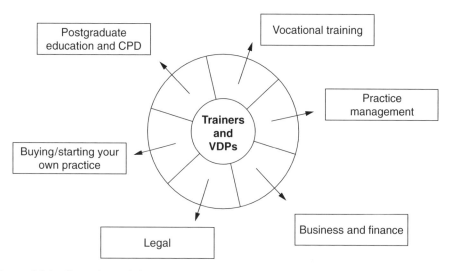

Figure A2.1 Overview of site content.

Appendix 3
Framework for tutorial discussions

The tutorial is the corner stone of the in-practice training programme. It involves active participation from the trainer and the VDP. For planning purposes, consider the tutorial to be made up of two elements: (1) the subject matter (content) and (2) the process, which can be linked in the following framework:

Stage 1	What are the priorities of the week? What are the topical issues? Is there anything important and/or urgent?
Stage 2	Where do you want to be?
Stage 3	What are your learning needs generally and in relation to (1) above?
Stage 4	Prioritise
Stage 5	What essential and desirable objectives will you focus on?
Stage 6	What tools (skills, resources, qualifications, opportunities) do you have?
Stage 7	What tools do you need?
Stage 8	How and when are you going to fulfil your learning objectives?
Stage 9	How will you know when you have achieved your objectives?

Examples of components and topics that may be relevant for a VDP.

Knowledge	Political awareness	Attitudes	Skills	Aspirations	Context	Legal requirements
Clinical	Policy	To other disciplines	Team working	Career	Settings	Health and safety
Information	Priorities	Patients	Communi-cation	Transferable skills	Population	Employment
Resources	Fashions	Lifelong learning	IT capability	Trainer	Networks	Revalidation
Experts	Change	Cultural	Practice development	Promotion	Practice priorities	Safe practice
Best practice			Specialisms Competent practitioner	Practice mission/ vision	Team relationships Historical service patterns	

Tutorial topics by content

This list contains some suggestions for tutorials. Some of the topics are very specific and will not take a complete hour, e.g. how to write a NHS prescription and related matters. Others are more involved and may take up more time, e.g. discussions about aesthetic dentistry. This list is not prescriptive and trainers are encouraged to use it as a prompt for further ideas and discussions.

Where possible, use the subject heading in the context of the working environment so it is perceived as relevant and real.

Law and ethics
• Current legislation
• Complaints procedures
• Role of Health Authority
• Health and Safety legislation

Dentistry in the NHS
6·8·03 • Organisation and structure of the NHS
• The future of the NHS: primary care groups/trusts

The practice
1·8·03 • Equipment and function
• Maintenance
1·8·03 • Organisational issues and management structure

The dental team
• Working with a dental laboratory
• Role of individual team members
• Guidelines on staff management

- Coping with interpersonal conflict
- Staff selection
- Motivation and reward
- Delegation
- The hygienist

Organisation and management
- NHS paperwork
- Record keeping
- The Dental Practice Board
- The Statement of Dental Remuneration
- Procedures for prior approval etc.
- The Dental Reference Service
- Referral protocol
- Prescriptions
- Private and NHS care options
- Fee setting

Clinical subjects
- Diagnosis and management
- Pain control
- Dealing with emergencies
- Periodontal therapy
- Tooth surface loss
- Treatment planning
- Aesthetic dentistry
- Provisional crowns and bridges
- Clinical photography
- Infection control
- Oral ulceration
- Antibiotics: use and abuse

Patient management
- Managing patient expectations
- The patient who refuses to pay
- Dealing with complaints
- Communication skills
- The nervous patient
- The high-risk patient

Practice management
- Understanding your payment schedule
- Practice systems
- Fee collection

- Security of records
- Use of IT
- Public relations and marketing

Financial management
- Cost control in general practice
- Associateships
- Keeping financial records
- Basic book keeping
- Banking and handling cash
- Choosing an accountant
- Other professional advisers

It will be helpful to both parties to try and keep records of the subjects that have been discussed. There are many ways that this can be done. In the example shown (Tables A3.1 and A3.2), the broad tutorial topics are listed on a spreadsheet which is divided so that it reflects six 10-minute time slots (the shaded region). Each time a subject is discussed for a minimum of 10 minutes, the trainer places a tick in the relevant shaded box. After a period of time, the spreadsheet will give a visual picture of what has been discussed and how much time has been spent on it. In the example shown, the total tutorial time is 4 hours and the spread of the subjects covered is easy to see at a glance. The reader can see that considerable time has been spent on practice/personnel introductions but very little information has been provided about the computer system (in this case because the nurse has responsibility for updating records). The emphasis on the tutorial subjects will vary from practice to practice according to practice circumstances.

This information can also then be recorded in a different format so that it reflects the chronological order of tutorial activity – *see* Table A3.3. In this case, a date entry for each tutorial is made and the trainer completes the category of subject matter discussed and covered, and the time spent on each. The headings reflect those used in Tables A3.1 and A3.2 but the information is presented in a different form. In the example shown, the date entry on 5.10.99 indicates that 20 minutes was spent discussing clinical issues, 30 minutes on administrative matters, 10 minutes on a practice management issue, 20 minutes on problem solving, and the type of activity that took place was a critical incident analysis. The timings are approximate but they do at least give a clear indication of the commitment that both trainer and VDP have to the process. The entire tutorial was in fact based on an incident involving a patient who had fractured the palatal cusp of a recently restored upper first molar, and the discussions around the various headings centred on this.

It should be emphasised that these spreadsheets are not prescriptive. Rather, they are ideas that trainers may want to consider or adapt for use in the training practice.

Table A3.1 Tutorial list

Tutorial topic		Comments
Orientation		
Practice overview	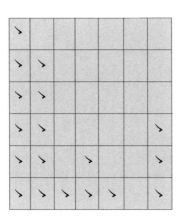	
Introduction to personnel		
Introduction to facilities		
Overview of surgery and basic maintenance		
Computer		
Concept of patient care		
Administration and paperwork		
Rules and regulations		
SDR	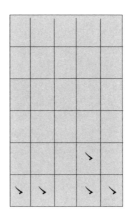	
NHS Regulations		
Dento-legal matters – consent/risk management		
Dental Practice Board		
Notes and record keeping		
Methods and materials		
Clinical techniques – overview	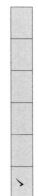	

Table A3.2 Tutorial list

Tutorial topic		Comments
Endodontics		
Simple restorative		
Advanced restorative		
Composites and glass ionomers		
Prosthetics		
Practice management		
Basics of finance		
Organisation and management systems		
HRM		
Efficiency and effectiveness		
Interpersonal communication		
NHS and independent care		
Payment systems		
Equipment maintenance and care		
Career development		
Associateship		

Table A3.3   Tutorial content by subject

Date	Clinical	NHS admin	Dento-legal	PM	HRM	Equip	PBL	Activity	Hands-on	Total time
5.10.99	20	30		10			20	C.I.A.		80
12.10.99										
18.10.99										
19.10.99										
26.10.99										
2.11.99										
9.11.99										
15.11.99										
16.11.99										
30.11.99										
7.12.99										
14.12.99										
15.12.99										
20.12.99										
21.12.99										

Useful tutorial structures

Some examples of useful structures which may help trainers in conducting tutorials are given below.

The GROW approach

The GROW technique is suitable for 15–30-minute interaction and can help VDPs to find a way forward with a problem (Middleton and Field, 2001).

G	goals	What would you like to achieve in this session? What needs to happen for you to achieve your aim? Will this be of real value to you? Is it a realistic aim?
R	reality	What is happening now? How often? When does it happen? Is this an accurate assessment? What effect does this have? What other factors are relevant? Who else is involved? What is their perception? What have you tried so far? (encouraging self-assessment)
O	options	What can you do? (all options) Who or what could help? Would you like suggestions? Which options interest you most? Why? What are the pros and cons? Rate the options 1–10 on practicality Would you like to choose one option now?
W	wrap up	What are the next steps? When will you take them? What might hinder your plans? What support do you need? How and when will you get it? How will you know you have achieved your goals?

The FRAME approach to planning educational objectives

F	few	Set one or only a few goals
R	realistic	These goals should be achievable
A	agree	If the process involves others, obtain their agreement
M	measurement	Ensure that you will know the goal has been achieved
E	explicit	Exclude hidden agendas and bias, and keep the process open

The POSSEER exercise

This is a helpful tool in assessing opportunities for behavioural change. It can help the VDP to identify a way forward using the processes outlined below.

P	positive	Make sure the goal is stated in positive terms, i.e. 'I'm always late' becomes 'I want to be on time'
O	owned	Define what is in the person's power to achieve, i.e. if you are always late because there is no public transport, then you can't catch an earlier bus
S	specific	Define the how, what, where, when and who
S	size	Make it a balance between possibility and challenge, i.e. not too small or too big
E	evidence	How will it be evident that the change has occurred? This needs to be explicit
E	ecology	How will the change fit into the person's wider existence?
R	resources	Are the tools for the job available?

Some observations on tutorials

In a recent study involving GP trainers, Caird and Ogden (2001) identified 20 'behavioural indices', which represented a range of possible teaching processes that took place during the one-to-one tutorial.

Trainers expressed their beliefs about what they believed to be a 'good tutorial'. The findings were ranked as follows:

1 Express opinion
2 Ask open questions
3 Provide facts
4 Check knowledge
5 Respond to enquiry
6 Prompt
7 Give information
8 Encourage
9 Challenge
10 Interpret
11 Be accepting
12 Ask for justification
13 Act as resource
14 Use silence
15 Share problem
16 Provide support
17 Criticise
18 Be non-judgemental
19 Disagree
20 Correct facts.

It was from this that the GP trainers identified their roles, as cited in Chapter 2 of this book.

Appendix 4
Reflections

This appendix has been written by a recent group of VDPs and is a summary of their perceptions of vocational training.

At the beginning

The prospect of leaving the secure environment of an undergraduate dental school to dive headfirst into general dental practice is a daunting experience at the very least. Two concerns dominate:

- how will we cope in the real world with no one there to check our work?
- how can we be sure that our work will be up to standard, that our cavity preparations will be caries free and our crown preparations are designed to the correct form and taper?

We are told that vocational training is the bridge, which will allow us to cross from the aspirations of the undergraduate environment to the challenges of general dental practice.

On reality

You cannot expect your trainer to check all your work, but you know that he/she is there if you run into any problems. Hands-on help is always available – this is reassuring. Make no mistake, you learn very quickly and learn what doesn't work. Experienced trainers in particular are good at helping out and correcting poor techniques.

Time is the enemy and we all feel that we are required to perform to high standards, but in a time efficient way. This is not easy. We are now beginning to recognise the limitations of our undergraduate curriculum in that it did not address aspects of working within the NHS. Working under the NHS requires a great deal of knowledge of what is and what is not permissible; most of us risk breaching regulations without even real-ising it. This is where VT helps – it teaches us the pitfalls of practice (the title of one of our earlier presentations!). We are constantly mindful of the responsibility we now have and the need to 'secure and maintain oral health' for our patients is always on our mind both from a clinical and medico-legal perspective.

On trainers

Well, they come in a variety of shapes, sizes and forms! Some are youth-ful and others ... well, let's just say less youthful. They have their individual personalities and quirks and some are genial and others more aggressive in their training style. One thing is certain – they are there to help and we value that. The relationship with your trainer depends on how you see them. Some VDPs see their trainer as a mentor or boss, but to others they are good drinking partners (we believe the technically correct word for this is 'friend'). We value the trainer's experience – they have seen it all before and we want to learn from that experience but we also learn to think for ourselves and there are occasions when our perspectives on a particular situation differ from that of the trainer. At undergraduate level that wasn't allowed – at this level it is! We are encouraged to think for ourselves and develop our own views and way of thinking. It happens slowly, but it happens.

On the study days

The year is made up of working in general practice and attending 30 study days during the year. The days are aimed at furthering your knowledge in both clinical subjects and in the areas of finance and prac-tice management. The study days are the best part of VT. We are reminded that it is a *study* day, but perhaps we could be forgiven for saying that it feels like a day off – which it is, a day off from practice! We thoroughly enjoy getting together with our peers and sharing expe-riences and concerns – we all agree that we shall miss this when it is all over. It is reassuring to learn that everyone experiences the same diffi-culties and that we can help each other by sharing these experiences. We also learn from each other because trainers approach problems in different ways.

The variety and content of the study days makes the year more inter-esting. We have away days to visit important institutions like the Dental Practice Board, participate in a range of hands-on courses, and visit the

BDA and the GDC. The BDA annual conference is excellent and the social event organised for all VDPs is a highlight.

The other days are held back at base and we are exposed to aspects of clinical dentistry, finance, practice management, medico-legal issues and career opportunities.

Occasionally, we get together and organise an extra-curricular activitiy. Our geographical base means that we are close to a greyhound racing stadium and we decide to all meet up one evening for a meal and an in-depth discussion on the merits of dog racing. For many of us, this is a first-time experience and something we shall look back on with amusement. We are given tips by people known in the trade as *'regular punters'* – we look upon this as a tutorial on *canine guidance*.

The year passes by very quickly. You find your clinical abilities improve and you feel more and more confident that you are able to handle difficult situations. Time management improves slowly and we are aware that we are becoming more efficient in our work methods.

VDPs tend to look to their VT adviser for help and guidance throughout the year. We know from talking to our peers that advisers are individuals and the course style and content is a reflection, to some extent, of their personality. Our adviser was very approachable, caring, knowledgeable and witty but above all else, we know he is someone we can approach in the future for advice and guidance. He will be happy to help.

On VT

VT is an ideal stepping-stone into general dental practice. We work in a comfort zone where we know the trainer will be there to help. It is an introduction to real world dentistry and although we start the year with little knowledge and understanding of the financial aspects of general practice, we feel more confident about these issues by the end of the year. The year helps us to decide whether general practice suits us.

We have some concerns and our collective experiences suggest that the process of VDP selection is perhaps not as fair and transparent as it should be. There is bias, and interviews openly reflect this bias. We would welcome an earlier publication date of approved practices so that it does not conflict with the stress of our final examinations, and it would be helpful if all regions published their lists at the same time.

In conclusion, it has been a fulfilling and enjoyable year. We have learned a great deal – probably more than we realise. The year has given us a wide exposure to all aspects of dentistry – clinical and managerial issues have been tackled. Experience is the best teacher. The course has now finished and, as we edit our contribution to this book on the very day we receive our certificates, we feel we have acquired the skills to progress to the next stage of our professional and career development.

Mr A Ahmed
Miss P Amin
Mr J Chauhan
Miss J Gibson
Miss H Lorimer
Mrs R Parkash
Miss B Patel
Miss S Usman
June 2001

Index